CW01506490

"This impressive collection of unpublishe with an exceptional opportunity to further influential thoughts and ideas of John Bow perspective on trauma and loss. This book is a must read for clinicians interested in the applications of attachment theory, for researchers who wish to broaden their understanding of attachment theory, and for developmental psychopathologists whose main principles have been greatly influenced by Bowlby's brilliant viewpoint. Professionals from a variety of disciplines, in addition to students in developmental and clinical science, will profit greatly from a thorough reading of this volume."

– *Dante Cicchetti,*
McKnight Presidential Chair, William Harris Professor,
Institute of Child Development, University of Minnesota, USA

"An extraordinary selection of previously unpublished material giving brilliant insights into the working of a brilliant mind. The editors are to be warmly congratulated on a collection that is not only of immense historical value, but remarkably speaks to current controversies in relation to trauma, resilience, and the philosophy of psychological science. An essential supplement to the Bowlby oeuvre."

– *Peter Fonagy,*
Professor & Head of the Division of Psychology
and Language Sciences at UCL; Chief Executive of the
Anna Freud National Centre for Children and Families, London, UK

"Attachment scholars and clinicians alike will find in this collection a series of rare treasures, among them insights into Bowlby's bold challenges to psychoanalysis and into the ways his work laid the groundwork for contemporary relational and trauma theory. These papers, many of them well over fifty years old, remind us – once again – of Bowlby's brilliance and remarkable prescience in predicting much of what is mainstream developmental and clinical theory today."

– *Arietta Slade,*
Clinical Professor at the Yale Child Study Center and Professor Emerita,
Clinical Psychology at the City University of New York, USA

"This book is a treasure. What a gift to have further seminal thoughts from one of the greatest thinkers of the twentieth century. Readers who want to know more about the scientist and those who want to know more about the clinician both will find this book valuable. All will enjoy learning more about the dogged curiosity and humility of this giant of a scholar. Bowlby was way ahead of his time in understanding segregated mental systems, developmental consequences of trauma, and family dynamics. He still speaks to us today about practical current issues such as displacement and migration."

– *Alan Sroufe,*
Professor Emeritus of Child Psychology, University of Minnesota, USA

"John Bowlby created a theory that enabled researchers and others to observe and ask questions about child-parent interactions in a completely new way. His theory laid the groundwork for studying how children and their parents construct an attachment relationship through sensitive and attuned interaction, what can go wrong in the process, and how attachment difficulties may be repaired. In a world in which people are increasingly distracted and alienated, attachment theory, as it has developed, offers the potential for promoting healing empathy, both for others and for oneself.

These newly published texts of John Bowlby are a treasure trove for anyone interested in attachment theory and its application to psychotherapeutic work."

– Prof. Dr. Med. Karl Heinz Brisch,
Chair of The Early Life Care Institute at the
Paracelsus Medical University, Salzburg, Austria

"This must-read volume re-affirms John Bowlby as a towering figure in psychological science. It shows how ahead of his time he was in his evaluation of the strengths and limitations of Freud's work (the essay on defences is a masterpiece), his encylopaedic command of ethological, psychological and neuroscientific evidence, and the brilliance and originality of his thought. Compiled by cutting-edge scholars, it reinforces Attachment, with its deep Darwinian roots, as an essential starting point for all serious psychologists, psychotherapists and mental health researchers."

– Prof Jeremy Holmes,
University of Exeter, UK

"John Bowlby was one of the most courageous and creative thinkers of the past century. He illuminated in unique ways the origins of our humanity. We are gifted here to have the privilege to understand further how he reflected on the central questions surrounding the early attachment relationship and wended his way towards his masterful trilogy on Attachment, Separation, and Loss. This volume of unpublished papers has many riches that will occupy Bowlby scholars and researchers long into the future."

– Karlen Lyons-Ruth, Ph.D., Professor,
Harvard Medical School, USA

"A fascinating insight into the workings of John Bowlby's creative mind, especially his prescient concerns about necessary future changes in psychoanalytic defence theory associated with traumatic loss of the mother in the earliest stages of human development."

– Allan N. Schore, Ph.D.,
Department of Psychiatry and Biobehavioral Sciences,
University of California at Los Angeles David Geffen School of Medicine, USA

Trauma and Loss
Key Texts from the John Bowlby Archive

During his lifetime, John Bowlby, the founder of attachment theory, was unable to publish as he wished due to strong opposition to his ideas. Now, with the support of the Bowlby family, several complete and near-complete works from the John Bowlby Archive at the Wellcome Collection are published for the first time.

The collection spans Bowlby's thinking from his early ideas to later reflections and is split into four parts. Part 1 includes essays on the topic of loss, mourning, and depression, outlining his thoughts on the role of defence mechanisms. Part 2 covers Bowlby's ideas around anxiety, guilt, and identification, including reflections on his observations of and work with evacuated children. Part 3 features three seminars on the subject of conflict, in which Bowlby relates clinical concepts to both political philosophy and psychoanalysis in innovative ways. Part 4 consists of Bowlby's later reflections on trauma and loss and on his own work as a therapist.

This remarkable collection not only clarifies Bowlby's relationship with psychoanalysis, but also features his elaboration of key concepts in attachment theory and important moments of self-criticism.

It will be essential reading for clinicians, researchers, and others interested in human development, relationships, and adversity.

Robbie Duschinsky is Senior University Lecturer in Social Sciences in the Primary Care Unit, University of Cambridge. He is also a Fellow and Director of Studies at Sidney Sussex College.

Kate White is an attachment-based psychoanalytic psychotherapist, supervisor, and member of The Bowlby Centre, London. She is also Editor Emeritus for *Attachment: New Directions in Psychotherapy and Relational Psychoanalysis* and Series Editor for The Bowlby Centre Monographs.

Trauma and Loss
Key Texts from the
John Bowlby Archive

Edited by Robbie Duschinsky and
Kate White

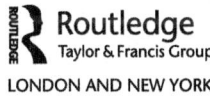
Routledge
Taylor & Francis Group

LONDON AND NEW YORK

First published 2020
by Routledge
2 Park Square, Milton Park, Abingdon, Oxon OX14 4RN

and by Routledge
52 Vanderbilt Avenue, New York, NY 10017

Routledge is an imprint of the Taylor & Francis Group, an informa business

British Library Cataloguing-in-Publication Data
A catalogue record for this book is available from the British Library

Library of Congress Cataloging-in-Publication Data
A catalog record has been requested for this book

ISBN: 978-0-367-34998-1 (hbk)
ISBN: 978-0-367-34999-8 (pbk)
ISBN: 978-0-429-32923-4 (ebk)

Typeset in Times New Roman
by Integra Software Services Pvt. Ltd.

Contents

Illustrations

Figures

Table

Acknowledgements

Our thanks go first to the Bowlby family and to Guy Dawson as chair of the trust holding the copyright to the papers in the John Bowlby Archive, in the Wellcome Collection. The family have enthusiastically supported our work to publish material from the Archive.

We are also very grateful to staff at the Wellcome Collection, especially Jenny Haynes and Ross MacFarlane, who have been most encouraging of this project and of public use of the Bowlby Archive. We would definitely encourage any reader of this book to explore the online catalogue for this archive and see what an inexhaustible, miraculous resource it is – and then to order material and visit the Wellcome Collection in Euston, London, to view it. We can guarantee a warm reception from the staff there.

We are also grateful to the Wellcome for their support for Robbie's research and especially for the Medical Humanities Investigator Award (Grant WT103343MA), which provided time for exploring the contributions of Bowlby and later studies of attachment to developmental science.

Our thanks also go to The Bowlby Centre for its support and financial commitment from the beginning. We are grateful to Jeremy Rutter, formerly chair of the Trustees, and to Mark Linington, formerly chair of the executive, for their encouragement and leadership.

Our thanks also go to Gareth Prosser, who is currently undertaking his clinical training at The Bowlby Centre and who has been our editorial assistant on this project. He has provided meticulous work on the texts, and we are very grateful for his involvement.

We are most grateful to our close colleagues and families who have been so supportive and who have provided affection and inspiration as we have worked.

Finally, a particular thank you to Elliott Morsia and his colleagues at Routledge.

Robbie Duschinsky and Kate White

Foreword

Miriam Steele and Howard Steele

Duschinsky and White have pulled together a treasure trove of unpublished writings of John Bowlby. Many of these rough gems foreshadowed Bowlby's published work, offering a deeper sense of his ideas and their development over time. Importantly, most of the papers here also offer sparkling and important insights beyond those available in Bowlby's published works.

This book adds to what we already know of Bowlby's thinking, with direct relevance to contemporary clinical work and prevailing concerns in society as a whole. We highlight below five chapters that contain distinctive hitherto unknown insights from the authoritative voice that conceived of attachment theory. In each chapter of the book, readers will find their own essential quotations to consider from these newly published words of John Bowlby. This is only a sampling:

1) Chapter 1 "Defences that Follow Loss". This monograph from 1962 presents valuable remarks on clinical phenomena, such as the meaning of coping and the origin of mental illness. In many respects, this is the "missing link" between psychoanalytic theory and attachment theory and will be of great interest to anyone interested in the interface between these two influential models of the mind. On display in this chapter, as in others in this volume, is Bowlby's consistent pride in the psychoanalytic enterprise and the determination he felt to clarify significant differences from his analytic teachers and colleagues (e.g., Freud, Klein).
2) Chapter 7 "Guilt and Family Contracts". This integration of psychoanalytic and legal theory offers ideas about promises and implicit contracts within families that will be of terrific interest to systemic practitioners, as well as others interested in the dynamics of family life. These reflections from the late 1930s are not available in Bowlby's published works.
3) Chapter 5 "Psychological Problems of Evacuation". Written around 1939–1942, this paper by Bowlby provides an evocative account of the effects of evacuation or separation from parents on children. Of particular

note is his attention to the unique effects of evacuation on infants and toddlers, as distinct from older children or adolescents.

4) Chapter 8 "A Psycho-Analytic Approach to Conflict and its Regulation". A paper presented at Stanford in 1958, this manuscript offers reflections relevant to both psychological and social conflict and specific remarks on how and when psychological conflict becomes relevant to clinical work.

5) Chapter 10 "Psychological Processes Evoked by a Major Psycho-Social Transition". This paper, presented at the Tavistock in 1974, offers add-itional comments on the deep emotional and cognitive work involved in the updating of internal working models (IWMs). In particular, Bowlby provides a compelling account of the inevitably slow and painful pro-cesses involved in changing core beliefs about the self, others and how to live, following "major psycho-social transitions" – what we may now typically refer to as loss or trauma. This is a reflection of the revolution in thinking about mental health in relational terms initiated by Bowlby.

This volume provides new information about the intellectual journey Bowlby followed in order to advance a new way of thinking about human psychological development that he would call "attachment theory". The close and deliberate attention Bowlby gave to the topics of separation from and loss of loved ones is in clear view in many of the chapters in this volume. His unique understanding of defensive processes deployed by the mind in the face of loss or trauma, or threats thereof, is also a great treat included in this volume. These are topics that remain of urgent relevance to research in developmental science and to the activities of those in the helping professions working with both children and adults. These papers deepen and add to our understanding of Bowlby's perspective and have much to say to discussions today about human psychology, child develop-ment, and clinical practice.

In the final chapter, Bowlby speculates about attachment theory in a talk given in 1985, only five years prior to his death, that, "Time only, and a great deal of further research, will tell whether it proves as promising as some believe or is merely leading to a blind alley. That is the way of sci-ence". Some thirty-five years on from this speculation, we can conclude that Bowlby's directive was far from a blind alley. On the contrary, he illu-minated the human need for close emotional relationships with some few people called family, the importance of the wider context that sustains and shapes these bonds, and the more-or-less complicated emotional journey we all follow as a function of how our close relationships fare.

Howard Steele & Miriam Steele, Professors of Psychology, and Co-Directors of the Center for Attachment Research, The New School for Social Research.

April 7, 2019, New York City

Introduction

Robbie Duschinsky and Kate White

This introduction will firstly provide the reader with a brief overview of Bowlby's theory about human relationships, followed by a discussion of the rationale for selecting these previously unpublished papers for this volume. Finally, we will give a short summary of the chapters and place them in the context of the wider Bowlby Archive. The summary draws out some ways that this previously unseen material is relevant to the caring professions.

The idea of attachment

> Intimate attachments to other human beings are the hub around which a person's life revolves, not only when he is an infant or a toddler or a school-child but throughout his adolescence and his years of maturity as well, and on into old age.
>
> (Bowlby, 1980, p.422)

An "attachment", in the term's technical sense, is an enduring relational bond with a few characteristic elements. One is that the other person is a "secure base", facilitative of exploration. Another is that the other person is a "safe haven", sought out for closeness and comfort especially under conditions of distress. Finally, anxiety is experienced when the other person is unexpectedly unavailable. Attachment relationships are especially visible in infancy. There attachment can be seen in the infant's tendency to seek and maintain physical closeness to a specific person or specific people especially when alarmed, distressed or ill.

John Bowlby also recognised our enduring need for others across the whole lifespan. When these relationships are going well, and those looking after us acknowledge and meet our needs for support and attunement in times of both stress ("safe haven") and enthusiasm ("secure base"), then we can explore the world with confidence.

John Bowlby, in collaboration with his colleague Mary Ainsworth, established that it was not only the physical proximity of our caregivers that was important but their relational and emotional availability to attune to our needs which was critical. They argued that the responsiveness of attachment figures to our distress in childhood, for example when becoming separated, would be related to our sense of self-worth and beliefs about the availability of others later in life. Through repeated interactions with our primary caregiver(s) we begin to learn what to expect from others and make predictions about what we can ask for and who we can emotionally depend upon.

With repeated responsive parenting it is suggested we develop an "internal secure base" the representation of which we can emotionally return to in times of alarm to regulate our inner state. This then can help us reach out to others for help. Just bring to mind the last time you found yourself alone and locked out of your home or you'd missed the last bus; maybe it was late and dark. Hopefully by using your mobile phone, you could reach a loved person "better able to cope with the world" than you could at that moment and who could help you. In the meantime, you might be able to calm yourself down by remembering other times when help came when you were frightened.

Bowlby's attachment theory

Bowlby first set out his initial ideas in works such as "The Influence of Early Environment in the Development of Neurosis and Neurotic Character" (1940), "Forty-Four Juvenile Thieves" (1944), and *Maternal Care and Mental Health* (1951). Through collaboration with exceptional colleagues such as James Robertson and Mary Ainsworth, these early ideas were then elaborated through empirical, observational research with young children who had been separated from their caregivers through hospitalisation (Bowlby et al., 1956; Bowlby et al., 1952). Subsequently, Bowlby's conceptualisation of the origins and nature of the attachment response was developed into attachment theory through a remarkable two-way dialogue from the mid-1950s with the expert in animal behaviour, Robert Hinde. Bowlby brought together ideas from clinical psychoanalysis with observations of animals, primates in particular, in theorising the function of the child's tie to familiar caregivers and its role within emotional development (Bowlby, 1957, 1958).

A commonly held position in the psychoanalytic theory of Bowlby's day was that mental health symptoms are ultimately caused by innate drives like sexuality and aggression. By contrast, Bowlby emphasised the significance of actual childhood experiences in shaping mental health. Furthermore, whereas psychoanalysts at the time often discussed ambivalence and contradictory feelings towards other people as innate to human beings, Bowlby emphasised that the acuteness and painfulness of such contradictions within us may well be shaped by our experiences of close relationships from childhood. He argued strongly against the commonly held idea that a child who showed distress regarding separation from the caregiver had been spoilt by too much affection. Instead, he proposed, distress on separation was part of the attachment response.

Bowlby was more concerned by the lack of distress shown by children who had been separated from their caregiver or caregivers for many months in the context of hospitalisation. He and collaborators observed that this lack of distress was associated with signals of a disruption of normative development, such as disorientation and "brittle" rage following the return of the child to the family (Bowlby, 1960). For well-supported children, however, these symptoms slowly turned into anxiety and depression, and for some, these symptoms too then ebbed. For others, however, the anxiety and depression contributed to difficulties in forming close relationships and developing what have become labelled by professionals as "conduct problems". Bowlby's understanding of these children with "difficult behaviour" was that their need for relational security over time had not been met and so "Through their eyes the world is seen as comfortless and unpredictable; and they respond either by shrinking from it or by doing battle with it" (Bowlby, 1973, p.208). Bowlby conceptualised the response of these young children as parallel, in important ways, to the grief response in adults and campaigned for young children to be permitted to receive visits by their caregivers when in hospital (Bowlby, 1961).

Bowlby's major theoretical statement setting out his ideas was the trilogy of books *Attachment* (1969), *Separation* (1973), and *Loss* (1980). In these works, Bowlby developed his theory of attachment into an account of mental health and ill health over the lifespan and a theory of human emotional life. Yet if Bowlby's published works are already available, what is the purpose of this book containing unpublished works? And why have the Bowlby family offered us their support for this project?

To this question we have three answers, which are interrelated. Firstly, Bowlby was not able to publish as he wished. From the first presentation to the psychoanalytic community in the 1940s, where he was ambushed and criticised aggressively by his colleagues, Bowlby was bruised and mindful of the hostility his ideas could generate. The engine-room of his thinking remained largely hidden from view and was thus protected from criticism and misunderstanding. This included a large number of unpublished works of theoretical speculations, as well as complete and incomplete articles and files upon files of notes and observations.

Secondly, the value of these previously unpublished texts lies in their potential for deepening and filling out our understanding of Bowlby's ideas. For instance, those who have read Bowlby's published works will know that the concept of "segregated systems" is among the most significant ideas in his later work: it receives a disorientingly short chapter in

Loss (1980), yet the concept organises much of the rest of the book and determines the direction of his thinking in his late essays (1988). Some subsequent attachment theorists have used Bowlby's short chapter in *Loss* on segregated systems as the basis for their thinking and design of measures of assessment (e.g., George & West, 2012). Yet researchers have been forced to extrapolate from a truncated account. The Bowlby Archive, however, reveals a short unpublished book on the subject from 1962 – eighteen years before the concept appears in print – entitled *Defences that Follow Loss: Causation and Function* (Chapter 1 of this volume).

A third justification lies in John Bowlby's consent for his papers to be deposited in the Wellcome Collection in London. From there, they are freely available to the interested public. Indeed, the John Mostyn Bowlby Archive (Bowlby Archive) is among the Wellcome's most popular collections. In our choice of papers for this volume, we have selected a fraction of those available. We have prioritised works that are largely complete, relate to the themes of trauma and loss, and contain material well beyond his published works in depth or scope in addressing a particular issue. We intend the volume to be a resource for those thinking about, appraising, and using attachment theory today. In an unpublished seminar delivered at the Tavistock Clinic in 1974 (PP/BOW/F.3/90), Bowlby noted that the appraisal, refreshment, and development of theories and models is best facilitated by "support and encouragement in tackling the task from a trusted companion". We hope that a conversation with John Bowlby's private reflections can facilitate consideration of the meaning and application of attachment theory today. Yet given the significant limits on what we could publish in a single volume, this book is also intended as a "film trailer" for the wider Bowlby Archive.

This book

The materials from the Archive in the present volume have been organised thematically around different aspects of the topic of trauma and loss and their consequences.

The first section of the book presents four theoretical texts by Bowlby. Chapters 1 and 2 are texts reflecting on loss and mourning. Bowlby appears to have suppressed them as too theoretically radical for the reading audience of the 1960s, though many of the ideas were eventually included in his later work. Part of the importance of these two chapters is that there is no other writing by Bowlby in which he is as explicit in the attempt to develop a general characterisation and theorisation of the nature of defence mechanisms. Bowlby critically discusses the work of Sigmund Freud, Melanie Klein, Anna Freud, and Helene Deutsch on mourning, revisiting their clinical cases. The two chapters also contain important reflections on aggression and despair as responses to loss and trauma, including aggression directed against the self. We have also included a letter from Mary Ainsworth to John Bowlby, offering him feedback on these ideas.

In addition to its value to researchers, the collection of previously unpublished papers gathered together in this book provides those who are working with people in distress with a wealth of ways to understand the often perplexing and difficult struggles we encounter in our caregiving and care-seeking roles. Further insight into Bowlby's theorising is illuminating and "experience-near". In particular, his extensive writing in the first two chapters on the way people keep themselves on an even keel through segregating overwhelming experiences, often related to loss, is particularly welcome. His emphasis on the level of segregation being at four different levels of intensity has a lot of resonance clinically. Noting that these processes are "beneficial in kind but faulty in amount", Bowlby continues:

> Defence is not conceived as being initiated in order to avoid some foreseeable consequence; and the ego is not credited with undertaking defensive measures for a purpose, either conscious or unconscious. Instead the individual is seen as the unwitting subject of processes that occur outside his awareness and for reasons that are unknowable to him.

In a humane and non-blaming way he encourages us to examine the cause, process, and function of defences including segregation, which he describes as being like "an iron curtain".

With this imagery, he helps us to understand the often perplexing difficulty we may have in permitting offers of support and love from new relationships because these contradict our entrenched forecasts that people cannot be trusted. A person who believes that they are unlovable leads them neither to expect support and help nor to recognize and respond to it when it is offered. Bowlby suggests that trusting a new relationship may also elicit a worry of being "in imminent danger of being abandoned". Thus an individual is compelled to maintain their isolated equilibrium in the safety of the "status quo".

Researchers and therapists who are interested in trauma and its links to the concepts of dissociation and disorganised attachment states of mind will find in this account much to illuminate their thinking and provide leads for further exploration.

Chapter 3 offers previously unseen reflections by Bowlby on the metapsychology of depression and mourning and the particular kinds of rumination associated with depressive cognition. In Chapter 4, Bowlby uses a discussion of Darwin's theory of emotions as a springboard for critical examination of the purposes of psychological classification. He raises the question – of much contemporary interest – regarding whether mental illness is best regarded as on a spectrum or categorically distributed. He applies these considerations to the concept of mourning.

The second section of the book presents three chapters addressing the themes of guilt, anxiety, and identification. Despite their status as early works, they are full of insights. For example, Chapter 5 presents Bowlby's reflections on the psychology of evacuation, with much of contemporary relevance, for instance in work with child refugees. He argues that every human being, from birth to old age, draws emotional sustenance and strength from those few people who constitute his home, a truth that will always need restating in a world often overwhelmed by economic stress and political strife. The text is full of practical advice for helping a child settle in a new environment, whilst also proposing the theory that it is the child who has felt unhappy and insecure at home who finds it most difficult to leave it. Bowlby documents, however, that, despite such individual differences, most children in the evacuation felt anxiety over the safety of parents and friends and that this was one of the principal causes of the outbreak of bedwetting documented in the early days of the evacuation. The distress of leaving home, the strangeness of new people, fears of doing the wrong thing, in a few cases a cool reception – all these could serve to make a child feel anxious, awkward, and uneasy. Yet Bowlby observes that where children are given a home, the evacuation experiences tended to be better than for those children who were billeted *en masse* in a big house.

Chapter 6 represents Bowlby's early attempt to wrestle with Freud's account of guilt and anxiety. Bowlby examines the role of different factors such as trauma and culture in shaping the tone and qualities of our moral reasoning. He then develops a revision of psychoanalytic theory in which the super-ego is conceptualised as operating in the name of preserving good social relations, whereas the ego-ideal serves the interests of achieving personal long-term aims. Bowlby also presents reflections on the idea of ego-phantasies: wishes the self has for the self.

The link between close relationships and morality is continued in Chapter 7, written a few years later. Here Bowlby develops a remarkable and innovative theory of anxiety and guilt through reflection on the implicit "contracts" made between family members. In Bowlby's account, a common pathway to unrealistic feelings of guilt is through contracts imposed by one party upon another. This leads him to a discussion of parental threats made to children, and the way in which love may come with implicit contracts attached. He observes that under the threat of losing the parent's love, a child may make the most ambitious promise, and argues that children feel guilty if they break this contract even if it was an imposed one and no guilt is realistically justifiable. Bowlby then goes on to consider contracts people may make with themselves and contracts the terms of which have become unconscious. He analyses the role of both in otherwise inexplicable feelings in adulthood.

Section three groups together three seminars delivered by Bowlby on the theme of conflict. The earliest, Chapter 8, develops a discussion of his therapeutic work with a woman experiencing deeply conflictual feelings about her mother. Bowlby theorises her illness as resulting from the unfavourable modes which she had adopted for regulating this painful conflict. Bowlby discusses his methodology for working with the patient to support the adoption of more favourable methods of regulation. This account allows him to illustrate his view that some intrapsychic conflict is inevitable and ubiquitous, but that the degree of conflict varies according to experience and that a major criterion for assessing a person's state of mental health lies in how they regulate intrapsychic conflicts. He argues that the therapist's task is to help all the different parts or "subsystems" within the person to become aware of the existence and nature of each other, to tolerate each other without too much anxiety and guilt, and to live with each other as parts of the total system.

The next seminar in this section, Chapter 9, brings together psychoanalytic theory and political philosophy in reflecting on the meaning of conflict and the ways in which potential conflicts can be best regulated in the clinical and political spheres. Speaking at Stanford University, during fellowships at the Center for Advanced Study, Bowlby and Ralf Dahrendorf discuss the nature of conflict, bringing together clinical concepts with ideas from political philosophy. They observe that conflicts can vary in their intensity, for example in the amount of energy spent by conflicting forces, the importance attached by these forces to certain issues, and the "cost" of victory or defeat. They also observe that conflicts can vary in the violence of their expression. Bowlby and Dahrendorf show the value in distinguishing clearly between the intensity and violence of a conflict. In clinical work as in politics, they argue that the minimum requirements of successful conflict regulation would seem to be a) recognition of the presence of conflict and of the true nature of conflicting forces, b) expression (if necessary, through organisations) of conflicting forces, and c) establishment of certain rules of the game to reduce the likelihood of violent conflict. The paper ends with a discussion of the concept of interdisciplinary research, its goals, and potential pitfalls.

The final text of the section, Chapter 10, is from some years later. Bowlby sets out to develop a general theory of different kinds of conflict, threading together ethology, psychoanalysis, and political philosophy within an overarching cybernetic framework. His basic premise is that where two or more messages reach us, we can only deal efficiently with one, even though we can monitor the others. He uses this model to reflect on how psychological conflicts may play out in shaping self-esteem and in pathways to depression. Applications are made to internal conflict and its impact on therapeutic relationships. Bowlby suggests that there is a potential to see that:

> The role of the psychoanalyst is that of mediator. His assistance is asked for voluntarily and accepted voluntarily. His task is to help all subsystems within the personality to become aware of the existence

and nature of each other, to tolerate one another without too much anxiety and guilt and to live with each other as parts of the total system, namely the personality itself.

The aim is, as it is in conflict resolution scenarios, to "increase communication and mutual understanding", in this case between the different parts of the self.

The fourth and final section offers two texts in which Bowlby looks back on his career and on how trauma and loss have been conceptualised. Both texts address Bowlby's work as a clinician. The first, Chapter 11, is a long autobiographical interview from the late 1970s. Bowlby's focus is on his involvement with the Child Guidance Clinic movement. The interview also considers the influence of his ideas on the social work profession, his relationship with Donald Winnicott and Robert Hinde and presents reflections on the relationship between the interests of clinicians and researchers. The final chapter of the book, Chapter 12, is a remarkable and candid account by Bowlby of his shortcomings as a therapist and the way in which these led him to feel the need to construct attachment theory. He compares his approach to that of Melanie Klein.

The wider Bowlby Archive

There is a huge array of materials in the Bowlby Archive beyond those included in the present volume. The present book can be no more than a trailer for this wider archive. We want to touch upon some of these, as we anticipate that providing this context will help the reader situate the texts included in this volume.

In his early twenties, Bowlby began his first attempts at scholarly work. In his first work, the 1929 "Essay on Experimental Education" (PP/BOW/A.1/19), Bowlby is already urging the need to bring a scientific approach to psychological questions and the need to recognise children's specific needs through a developmental perspective. He states that:

> This essay has for its purpose the recommendation of experiment in education and evaluation ... and the results of their practice tested in a scientific spirit and that forcing children only to satisfy adult tendencies is to overlook the fact that if these childish impulses remain unsatisfied they are very likely to interfere with the development and satisfaction of adult ones.
>
> (Bowlby, 1929)

A highlight of the Bowlby Archive is the vast array of notes and reflections made as Bowlby read and reflected on psychoanalytic ideas. In 1933, he registered as a PhD student at University College, London. Initially, the title for his PhD research was the "Interrelation of Sexual and Aggressive Impulses". In the Archive are his notes from 1933–1936 as he worked intensively on elaborating his account of human motivation, against the backdrop of the psychoanalytic ideas of his time. Laying the ground for his later concept of "working models", Bowlby considers how the ego comes to "contain within itself representation of the external world in the shape of verbal and visual symbols".

Representations of close relationships are independent from but influence representations which can be of the self or the world in general, as children "rapidly acquire working rules not only as to how all human beings behave, but also how individuals behave" (PP/BOW/D.1/2/10). It was in this era that Bowlby composed a number of handwritten, unpublished theoretical papers, among them "Freud and the Super-Ego" (Chapter 6 in this volume) and, a little later, a manuscript on guilt and implicit contracts within families (Chapter 7).

An era of Bowlby's life that had a lasting impact but which has to date been almost invisible in the published record has been his activity during World War II, during which he worked as an army psychiatrist in a variety of roles. The Bowlby Archive contains a large range of materials relating to these years. For instance, there is his contribution to the Cambridge Evacuation Survey, reporting on difficulties experienced by children (PP/BOW/C.5.4/2). We have included here Bowlby's unpublished essay "Psychological Problems of Evacuation" (Chapter 5), written during this period. However, in the Archive there are very many other texts from the war years.

One example is the 1940 Bowlby and Soddy "War Neurosis Memorandum" (PP/BOW/C.5/1), justifying the value of psychotherapy rather than punishment for traumatised war veterans suffering from "shell shock". Bowlby and Soddy document symptoms including "amnesias, confusional states, transient psychoses, anxieties, depressions, dreams and panic states, trance states, severe tics, inhibitions". Considering their cases, Bowlby and Soddy observe that:

> there is, of course, a group of patients who make steady progress when treated by rest, sedatives and occupations without any psychotherapy. There is, however, another group whose emotional disturbance is deep seated, who suffer from amnesia of shocking experiences and who, in the view of many authorities, require psychotherapy.

The cause of this emotional disturbance was conceptualised as a "conflict fear versus duty", in which the symptoms represented the mental fallout of a sustained period in which this conflict was intense and unresolved. Bowlby and Soddy argued that continuity of care is crucially important in supporting patients through the disorientation, then anxiety and depression, that has stemmed from their traumatic experiences:

Patients should as soon as possible be sent to a centre where they can be adequately looked after in all their phases from the confusional state through the anxiety and depression which follows, to convalescence. For a man to be moved from one hospital to another, or from the care of one medical officer to another during the course of his illness is bad psychotherapy and liable to promote a chronic condition.

Looking back on his career, in a 1984 letter to Phyllis Grosskurth (PP/BOW/A.5/7) Bowlby wrote that the war gave him time to develop his ideas and evidence of the importance of real life events. Before the war, he felt he would not have been ready for open conflict with the established psychoanalytic orthodoxies of his day. After the war, he was. The Bowlby Archive contains the important "Public letter to Melanie Klein" (PP/BOW/G.1/4), unpublished but circulated around the Institute of Psycho-Analysis, following the presentation of Klein's paper "A Study of Envy and Gratitude" to the Institute in 1956. Bowlby begins the letter by acknowledging that, "I have, since before the war, been profoundly influenced by your insistence on the central importance of the conflict of ambivalence for the loved object starting early in life, and all my own thinking stems from that."

However, Bowlby disagrees with Klein's account of innate drives and her assumption that a child's ambivalence towards caregivers is a matter of phantasy, little shaped by actual experiences. Bowlby states that:

I am afraid I have much difficulty in accepting your view that envy first develops in the first few months of life because I think it rather unlikely that cognitive functioning is adequate for it to occur before, say, twelve months or even later... Piaget's work on the construction of the object suggests to me that these rather complicated cognitive processes are unlikely to be developed much before the first birthday.

Klein's reply is also available:

If I were to reply to your letter in detail, as it would necessitate, it would take up a good deal of my time, because actually you have touched on fundamentals on which my whole work is based. The fact that the unconscious of the child, his impulses, and his desires, are operative long before he has acquired the functions you refer to, is one of the tenets of my whole work.

Other major highlights of the Bowlby Archive are the detailed observations of hospitalised children made by James Robertson within Bowlby's research group. The Archive contains drafts preparing for a book on the subject. This work was ultimately not published, in part due to personal differences between Bowlby and Robertson and in part due to theoretical differences between the authors in how to interpret the observations (Van der Horst & Van der Veer, 2009). Bowlby's own reflections were elaborated to some extent in published articles such as "Separation Anxiety" (1960). However, they were most fully elaborated in two significant unpublished works of theory (Chapters 1 and 2 of the present volume). In Robertson's meticulous documentation of individual cases of human suffering, the foundation of core elements of Bowlby's later theory become clear. For instance, the importance of reunion experiences as an index of mental health was discovered, a finding that would be consequential for Mary Ainsworth's later research using brief separations to study individual differences in attachment. For instance, in a manuscript in the Bowlby Archive (PP/BOW/D.3/11–12), the case of Alex is described:

> Alex's initial response to reunion with his mother was surprising. It showed the same ready affectionate response to his mother that was found otherwise only in a few of the children ... who had fretted for their mothers throughout separation, and were inferred to have maintained a dependency relationship with them despite the breach in continuity. On the other hand it seems certain that Alex did not go through a phase of overdependency after reunion ... He seemed very much the same with respect to the looseness of ties with other people as he had been before separation. Since Alex is the only child who had really bad relations with his mother before separation, it is impossible to know whether or not his behaviour is typical of such children. ...
>
> She had little time for him and indeed did little for him when she had time. It seems safe to infer that even before separation she rejected him in her underlying attitude as well as in the fact of her neglect, for she expressed regret that she had not placed him in an institution. ...
>
> It would seem that neglected and rejected children would have patterns and sequences of response to separation and reunion differing from those manifested by children with normal pre-separation child-mother relations.

The Archive also includes an extraordinary number of transcripts and notes of papers delivered as talks but not worked up or only excerpted in published works. These texts allow a reader to see Bowlby thinking about issues in more depth than he gives in the published works and a selection has been included in the present volume (Chapters 4, 8, 9 and 10). The Archive permits a reader to be included as part of the audience in Bowlby's historic seminars – for example at Stanford University, the British Psychological Society, or the interdisciplinary workshops held by Bowlby at the Tavistock Clinic.

The Archive also contains materials that ended up "on the cutting room floor". With some of the material, it is clear that it was excluded on the grounds that it was of less scientific interest. However, some of the exclusions are exceptionally interesting. "The Place of Defensive Exclusion in Depressive Disorders" forms Chapter 3 of the present volume and was a chapter drafted for *Loss* (1980). We suspect that it was excluded to make an already long book a little shorter, though the exact reason is unknown. In other cases, the reason for the exclusion appears to have been theoretically motivated, for example, a chapter on "Distress at Loss of Home" (PP/BOW/H.55) that was cut from *Separation* (1973). Bowlby was keen in this book to emphasise the distinction between other mammals who have a burrow for protection and human infants who require a relationship with an older human in order to survive.

Though the chapter on attachment to a place was excluded from *Separation* (1973), Bowlby nonetheless elsewhere in the book assumes that humans form attachments to particular loved places. The result is an ambiguity about the appropriate extension of the attachment concept. This ambiguity has had significant consequences for those inheriting Bowlby's ideas. For instance, there has been heated debate about whether attachment to religious figures is an acceptable extension of Bowlby's theory (Granqvist, 2010). Criticisms have been levelled at Bowlby for contributing to a lack of concern with familiar places when children are moved in adoption and fostering decisions informed by attachment theory (Jack, 2008).

Finally, the Archive also contains important retrospective documents, as Bowlby looked back on his long career. Among these are Chapters 11 and 12 of the present volume. There are many others though in the Archive. One is the 1979 manuscript "The Ten Books Which Have Most Influenced My Thought" (PP/BOW/A.1/8). In this account, for example, Bowlby describes first reading Freud's *Introductory Lectures on Psychoanalysis* in 1928 as an undergraduate at Cambridge. In 1929, "when I worked briefly at a school for disturbed children", Freud's work "came alive for me ... and has been a major influence on all my later work". Also of interest is Bowlby's description of encountering Thomas Kuhn's (1962) *The Structure of Scientific Revolutions*. "I read this probably in 1964 when the paperback edition came out. It has had a profound influence on my whole conception of what science is and how scientists operate". Another significant retrospective text is the 1986 interview with the BBC (PP/BOW/F.5/8). Here, for example, we learn about the origins of the link Bowlby proposed between early experiences of very extended separation and children's difficulties in regulating their feelings and behaviour:

> That started in I suppose in 1937 or 1938. I was seeing children at the London Child Guidance Clinic and I happened to see two cases, one after another, in which each of these children who had been referred because they were so-called incorrigible, they were stealing and

generally speaking being very difficult and each of them had spent nine months in a hospital when they were eighteen months old. In those days children who got a fever were whipped off to an isolation hospital, they stayed there for such time as was necessary... parents weren't allowed to visit in those days and when they returned home at the age of two years and three months they were remote, emotionally remote... with their parents. It was striking that these two stories, one of them was a little boy, the other a little girl – these stories were extraordinarily similar.

Conclusion

Already a decade ago, standing out against the general turn away from theory within psychology, attachment theory was considered one of the last big paradigms standing in the area of child development: "The Bowlby-Ainsworth tradition is a rare example of a more general or 'grand theory' that makes predictions about behaviour and emotion across multiple domains of psychological functioning and across the life span" (Waters & Cummings, 2000, p.164). Today, attachment theory not only forms the basis of an international research programme but has attracted a widespread clinical audience and achieved renewed salience with the "neurological turn" in policy and public discourse about childhood. Simons (2014) has argued against the need for theory within psychology, as "accumulated evidence for reliable effects is the lasting legacy of science – theories come and go" (Simons, 2014, p.79). Yet a well-founded theory like attachment theory, based on and extended by accumulated evidence, is useful. It can help researchers and clinicians organise experience, tolerate uncertainty, come to insights, make plans, and can support the flow of ideas between different domains, such as between clinical work and research.

We are honoured and delighted to bring to publication these papers which extend and enrich our understanding of what it is to be vulnerable and human in the twenty-first century. We are grateful to the Bowlby family for their permission to make them available and to the staff at the Wellcome Collection who have cared for and preserved these materials and who are so enthusiastic when people come to visit and encounter them.

References

Bowlby, J. (1940). The influence of early environment in the development of neurosis and neurotic character. *The International Journal of Psycho-Analysis, 21*: 154–178.

Bowlby, J. (1944). Forty-four juvenile thieves: Their characters and home-life. *The International Journal of Psycho-Analysis, 25*: 19–53.

Bowlby, J. (1951). *Maternal Care and Mental Health*. Geneva: World Health Organisation Report.

Bowlby, J. (1957). An ethological approach to research in child development. *British Journal of Medical Psychology, 30*: 230–240.

Bowlby, J. (1958). The nature of the child's tie to his mother. *The International Journal of Psycho-Analysis, 39*: 350–373.

Bowlby, J. (1960). Separation anxiety. *The International Journal of Psycho-Analysis, 41*: 89–113.

Bowlby, J. (1961). Processes of mourning. *The International Journal of Psycho-Analysis, 42*: 317–340.

Bowlby, J. (1969). *Attachment and Loss, Vol I, Attachment*. London: Hogarth Press.

Bowlby, J. (1973). *Attachment and Loss, Vol II, Separation: Anxiety and Anger*. London: Hogarth Press.

Bowlby, J. (1980). *Attachment and Loss, Vol III, Loss: Sadness and Depression*. London: Hogarth Press.

Bowlby, J. (1988). The role of attachment in personality development. In: J. Bowlby, *A Secure Base, Clinical Applications of Attachment Theory* (pp. 134–154). London: Routledge.

Bowlby, J., Ainsworth, M., Boston, M., & Rosenbluth, D. (1956). The effects of mother-child separation: A follow-up study. *British Journal of Medical Psychology, 29*: 211–247.

Bowlby, J., Robertson, J., & Rosenbluth, D. (1952). A two-year-old goes to hospital. *Psycho-Analytic Study of the Child, 7*: 82–94.

George, C. & West, M. (2012). *The Adult Attachment Projective Picture System*. New York: Guilford.

Granqvist, P. (2010). Religion as attachment: The Godin award lecture. *Archive for the Psychology of Religion, 32*: 5–24.

Jack, G. (2008). Place matters: The significance of place attachments for children's well-being. *British Journal of Social Work, 40*: 755–771.

Kuhn, T. (1962). *The Structure of Scientific Revolutions*. Chicago: University of Chicago Press.

Simons, D. J. (2014). The value of direct replication. *Perspectives on Psychological Science, 9*: 76–80.

Van der Horst, F. C. & Van der Veer, R. (2009). Separation and divergence: The untold story of James Robertson's and John Bowlby's theoretical dispute on mother–child separation. *Journal of the History of the Behavioral Sciences, 45*: 236–252.

Waters, E. & Cummings, M. (2000). A secure base from which to explore relationships. *Child Development, 71*: 164–172.

Part I

Mature theoretical writings

Chapter I

Defences that follow loss

Causation and function

February, 1962. [Editors: Wellcome Collection Archive PP/BOW/D.3/78]

Introduction

In the preceding paper[1] (Bowlby, 1960) the conclusion was reached that defensive processes, such as repression, splits in the ego, and denial, are readily initiated in a young child during separation from his mother-figure. Examination of the twin problems of what causes these defensive processes to be initiated and what functions, if any, they serve was, however, postponed. This was because they are the central problems of any theory of defence and so of psycho-analysis itself. "The theory of repression", Freud insisted, "is the corner-stone on which the whole structure of psycho-analysis rests" (Freud, 1914d, p.16).

Largely because in this enquiry I have adopted a theory of motivation different from the traditional one, the theory of defence that I shall advance is different also. Inevitably this has far-reaching consequences, not least for the theory of mental structure. This paper, therefore, takes us into the heart of meta-psychology. Moreover, despite the task in hand being limited to defences that follow loss, to confine the discussion to such defences is not possible. The defences in question, especially repression and splitting, are so central to any theory of defence that time and again we are faced with basic problems in the general theory.

The paper falls into three parts. In the first I shall examine some main features in the general theory of defence, including the phenomena to which it is habitually applied and the way in which the problems of the causation and function of defence are usually approached. Principal aims are to lay bare the nature of the data that require explanation and to draw attention to some of the difficulties posed by traditional theory. One such is the contradiction that confronts the type of theory that, whilst recognising that immaturity is particularly conducive

---

1 [Editors' note:] We suspect this is J. Bowlby (1960).

to defence, postulates the existence of a considerable degree of mental organization before the defence can occur.

I shall also indicate some of the points at which the theory I am advancing resembles the traditional ones, especially Freud's concept of primary repression arising from trauma. This concept was present in his early work and again after 1926. He developed it as a response to his recognition that, so far from being the result of repression, anxiety is a principal condition from its onset, and that, moreover, "the earliest outbreaks of anxiety, which are of a very intense kind, occur before the super-ego has become differentiated" (Freud, 1926d, p.94).

In the second part I shall concentrate on the particular problems presented by the tendency for defensive processes to be evoked after a loss has been suffered. Here I draw both on direct observations of the way young children respond during a separation and also on data obtained in the course of the analysis of older subjects, such as was reported in an earlier paper on *Pathological Mourning and Childhood Mourning* (Bowlby, 1963). The mental state arising, it is held, is characterised mainly by the co-existence of two contradictory motivational systems, which are in some way segregated from one another. The problem, therefore, is to understand the nature of the segregating process, the conditions that cause it to take the particular form it does after a bereavement, and the functions that in health the segregation processes serve. The hypothesis advanced is one that enables us to view psychological illness in the same light that Claude Bernard (1865, 1961), taught us to view psychological illness, namely as the outcome of processes that are beneficial in kind but faulty in amount. Defence is not conceived as being initiated in order to avoid some foreseeable consequence; and the ego is not credited with undertaking defensive measures for a purpose, either conscious or unconscious. Instead the individual is seen as the unwitting subject of processes that occur outside his awareness and for reasons that are unknowable to him. Although, perhaps, he may come later to explain and support his behaviour by plausible rationalisations, the true causes of it lie, it is held, far beyond his world of reason. Thus it is an hypothesis as applicable to animals as to man.

Concepts of defence

Defensive behaviour and defensive process

As Sperling (1958) has pointed out, when a list is made of the phenomena that are habitually termed defences the items on it are heterogeneous in nature. The term indeed has been applied to phenomena as widely variant as disease entities, character, symptom complexes, affects, physiological states and processes, psychological states and processes, art forms, and behaviour of both social and anti-social kinds. From this array it is useful to select two main usages which appear central for the discussion of causation and function.

One main usage refers defence to psychological processes, such as repression. Logically such processes have the status of inferences, since they cannot be directly observed. Nevertheless, they are inferences only one step removed from observation and therefore can readily be related to observed data. It is in this sense that Freud (1894a) first proposed the concept and himself used it; and it has been in regular use in this way ever since.

The other common usage refers to certain forms of behaviour, with their associated affects and fantasies which are grouped together because they seem to have something in common. Examples are obsessional rituals, manic behaviour, attacking one's own shortcomings in others. As forms of behaviour, they are open to immediate observation. Since, in addition, they (or verbal reports about them) are our basic data, it is wise to start the discussion with them.

On examination it seems that the different forms of *defensive behaviour* belong to at least three different classes. The simplest class comprises behaviour which is unchanged except that it is diverted from one object to another.[2] A second class comprises reaction formations, the basic nature of which is an accentuation of one type of behaviour in place of another type, a strong potential for which, though in great part inactivated, can be inferred. Reaction formations include both behaviour of an excessively polite, cleanly or ascetic kind and also behaviour of an excessively truculent, hostile or promiscuous kind. A third class, which is heterogeneous, comprises behaviour which is neither unchanged in form, as in displacement, nor the opposite of something else, as in reaction formation. It includes behaviour commonly referred to as regressive, e.g. thumb-sucking or masturbation following a disappointment, and also behaviour of other types, such as, for example, the care of a vicarious figure following loss. The theories I believe worth exploring to account for this third class are those advanced to account for what the ethologists have termed "displacement activity".

The notion lying behind the grouping together as defensive of these three classes of behaviour (and their associated affects and fantasies) is that the behaviour in question appears to be an alternative to behaviour of another kind which is more *appropriate* to the situation and which may be manifested concurrently, albeit only in covert and fragmentary ways. Whilst a potential for both sorts of behaviour is always present, the one that is less appropriate has dominance and is described as defensive.

It will be noted that in referring to different sorts of behaviour I have each time added in brackets "with its associated affects and fantasies". The reason is that I conceive overt behaviour to be only one component of

---

2 [Bowlby notes:] In psycho-analytical terminology "displacements"; in ethological terminology "redirected" activities.

a motivational system[3] within the organism, and fantasies, thoughts and affects, conscious and unconscious, to be integral to, and other components of, such systems. This usage calls for a note of explanation.

In a previous paper (Bowlby, 1961)[4] I drew attention to the difficulties that arise in theory construction when, instead of behaviour of a particular kind directed towards a particular object or goal, affect is taken as the main class of datum. There it was seen how, in studies of mourning, pre-occupation with the affects of grief and guilt had led to the urge to recover the lost object and to reproach it for its desertion both to be neglected. Once the nature of the motivated behaviour is recognised, on the other hand, the place of affects are found to be more easily understood. The same advantage is held to obtain when defence is approached from the standpoint of behaviour and motivation.

The simpler the organism the shorter the route between motivation system and action; the more developed the organism the greater the number of add-itional systems interposed between them. Although in man the processes arising in these intermediate systems are very complex and may result in long delay between an *urge* to act and action and also to great transformation between the act originally motivated and the one finally taken, the intermediate processes themselves are no more than links in a chain[5] that connects a motivational system with overt behaviour. It is in terms of motivational systems and motiv-ated behaviour, therefore, that they are best understood. From this standpoint ordered thought and day-dream are both conceived as forms of trial action; and unconscious phantasy as a form of trial action at an unconscious level. Similarly defensive fantasy, such as day-dreams of success, is conceived as a special and latent form of defensive behaviour.[6]

Let us now turn to *defensive processes*. They can best be defined as those processes within the organism that create barriers to interaction between different motivational systems. In the ordinary way interaction between systems is free. For example, there are commonly next to no barriers between, say, the systems governing a man's domestic behaviour, his

---

3 [Bowlby notes:] A motivational system is conceived as the product of the integration of a number of what I have termed instinctual response systems. For example, whilst clinging and following are each the manifestation of particular instinctual response systems, the resulting attachment behaviour to a special figure is conceived as the manifestation of a motivational system composed of these and other instinctual response systems, each of which (through learning) has come to have the presence of the figure as its consummatory situation.

4 [Editors' note:] We think this is J. Bowlby (1961).

5 [Bowlby notes:] A more accurate figure of speech might be "nodes in a network".

6 [Bowlby notes:] Insofar as I use the term "behaviour" in this rather broad way, I follow Rapa-port: "Behaviour in this theory is broadly defined, and includes feeling and thought as well as overt behaviour". The model of the mental apparatus is in keeping with that of modern phil-osophy (e.g. Hampshire, 1962). [Editors' note:] Likely this is D. Rapaport (1953) and S. Hampshire (1962).

professional behaviour and his vacation behaviour. Although each may be organised in a way that is very different from the others, they contain common elements, there are no striking incompatibilities, and in a fairly ordered way each governs behaviour during appropriate periods. The requirements of each are communicated to the others and when they conflict, as habitually they do, regulation is tolerably smooth and efficient.

When defensive processes are present, on the other hand, each system seems divorced from the others and at war with them. As a result, one or more dominate the scene whilst the others influence behaviour only in a furtive and fragmented way; conflicts and contradictions remain unregulated so that behaviour stemming from one sometimes cancels behaviour stemming from another. Often the subject is unaware or only partially aware of the existence of some of them. It is a state of affairs that was summed up by Freud in the *Outline* in the following words: "indeed a universal characteristic of the neuroses [is] that there are present in the subject's mental life, as regards some particular behaviour, two different attitudes, contrary to each other and independent of each other" (Freud, 1940a [1938], p.77). It is to the processes that lead these "attitudes", or motivational systems as I am terming them, to be independent and segregated from each other that the concept of defensive process is best applied.

It thus appears that the term defence is habitually used to refer (a) to behaviour (with its associated affects and fantasies) that is in some way alternative to and co-existent with another sort of behaviour (with its associated affects and fantasies), and (b) to the psychological processes that are held to be responsible for this other sort of behaviour not being manifested in an open and direct way. Although this double usage is confusing, in it lies the essence of defence. The concept of defence is invoked both to describe and also to explain a condition of the organism in which at least two motivational systems are not only both of them active (or potentially so) but are so segregated from one another by some kind of barrier that the usual processes by which incompatible motivational systems are regulated are unable to operate. It is in order to distinguish these two usages that I speak on the one hand of "defensive behaviour" and on the other of "defensive process". The traditional terms "defence mechanism" and "method of defence" do not make this distinction and are therefore unsatisfactory.[7] The many other phenomena to which the term defence is applied need individual examination. Many of them, e.g. physiological and psychological states and processes, in this theory fall into the category of consequences, often pathological consequences. The problem that now confronts us is how best to understand these processes and the conditions that give rise to them. Let us look next at how Freud and other analysts have approached it.

---

7 [Bowlby notes:] For example the list of defence mechanisms given by Anna Freud (1936, p.47) includes both defensive process, e.g. repression, and defensive behaviour, e.g. reaction formation.

Primary and secondary repression

A reading of Freud's accounts of defensive processes shows that he distinguishes two main classes. One class he conceives as operating at a comparatively low psychological level, the second at a higher one. Sometimes he stresses the one and sometimes the other: both are described in his final work, the *Outline* (Freud, 1940a [1938]). "For two different reasons," he there remarks, "the id is the source of ... dangers" against which the ego has to defend itself. "In the first place, an excessive strength of instinct can damage the ego in the same way as [can] an excessive 'stimulus' from the external world"; it does so by destroying the ego's dynamic organisation. In this hypothesis neither learning processes nor foresight are implied. Instead, the danger is conceived as that of the direct disruption of ego organisation by excess excitation arising from the id, and the defensive process as being called into play automatically to prevent its happening. "In the second place," he continues, "experience may have taught the ego that the satisfaction of some instinctual demand that is not in itself unbearable would involve dangers in the external world, so that an instinctual demand of that kind itself becomes a danger." (Freud, 1940a [1938], p.73). According to this hypothesis instinctual demand is curtailed because, through painful experience, the individual has learned that unfavourable consequences follow satisfaction.

In *Inhibitions, Symptoms and Anxiety* (Freud, 1926d), in which he first clearly drew the distinction, Freud termed the first process "primary repression". In keeping with this, we may term the second process "secondary repression", though Freud himself does not seem to have done so.

From this description it is clear that the two sources of danger and anxiety Freud postulates are radically different from one another, and that the *same holds* for the two kinds of defensive process that he believes to have been evoked. Freud's *second* source of danger is readily intelligible. Not infrequently our actions meet with ill-results, either from the physical world – fire burns us – or from the social – people dislike being ill-used and retaliate. In the course of experience, therefore, we learn gradually to control our actions, albeit only imperfectly; impetuous acts stemming from the urgent promoting of instinctual drives[8] can still lead us into trouble. As a consequence, the instinctual drives are themselves sensed as dangerous. The nature of Freud's *first* source of danger, on the other hand, is much less obvious. How are we to understand his idea that excess of excitation may endanger ego organization? If this is indeed a danger against which defences are required, it seems evident they will be defences of a kind very different to those required to guard against the second source of danger.

---

8 [Bowlby notes:] Rapaport adopts "instinctual drive" for the translation of Freud's "trieb". [Editors' note:] This is likely to be D. Rapaport (1953).

It is in fact my thesis that for psychopathology the first source of danger and the types of defence that it evokes is of far more consequence than is the second source of danger and the types of defence it evokes. The principal reason for thinking so is that the theory of primary repression fits far better than does that of secondary repression the evidence regarding the phase of ontogeny during which pathological defences are most apt to occur.

Empirically, there is good reason to believe that defensive processes of a pathological kind are particularly apt to be evoked in infancy – the more immature and therefore less differentiated the mental organisation, it seems, the more likely. This faces the theory of secondary repression with a major difficulty, because, as Freud himself realised (Freud, 1915d, p.147), it predicates a considerable degree of mental organization before repression can occur. The theory of primary repression by contrast predicates no such thing. On the contrary it was explicitly constructed by Freud after his recognition that defence is evoked by anxiety and to comply with his belief that the "earliest outbreaks of anxiety, which are of a very intense kind, occur before the super-ego has become differentiated" (Freud, 1926d, p.94). In the same way, the theories of defence advanced by Fairbairn (1952) and Melanie Klein (1952) are each designed to take account of this. The theory that I shall sketch is of this type.

The critical idea underlying Freud's concept of primary repression is that of trauma. In the course of his theorising[9] this idea had a checkered career. At first it was in favour, indeed alone. In the preliminary communication of hysteria by Breuer & Freud (1893a) trauma is the pathogen and the initiator of defence. Thus, in the paragraph in which the word "repression" is first used, reference is made to patients who "have not reacted to a psychical trauma because the nature of the trauma excluded a reaction" (Freud, 1893a, p.10). "The psychical trauma – or more precisely the memory of the trauma – acts like a foreign body which long after its entry must continue to be regarded as an agent that is still at work" (Freud, 1893a, p.6). In the following year the theory Freud elaborates in *The Neuro-Psychoses of Defence* (Freud, 1894a) has as its central feature the notion that symptoms arise because the psychic apparatus is unable to deal with too much of "something which possesses all the attributes of a quantity ... a quota of affect or sum of excitation" (Freud, 1894a, p.60).

A little later, however, after his disillusionment over the reality of sexual seduction, he lost confidence for a time in the traumatic theory of pathogenesis. His recognition, moreover, of the almost ubiquitous influence of unconscious motivation, which he was exploring in the following decade in

---

9 [Bowlby notes:] In tracing this history I am much indebted to C. Brenner (1957).

connection with dreams (Freud, 1900a), everyday life (Freud, 1904b) and jokes (Freud, 1905c), led his interest away from psychopathology. Processes arising from maturational and cultural influences now stole his attention and the second concept of repression was born. So far indeed did he in the next two decades come to identify himself with the concept that repression derives from awareness of unfavourable consequences of action that in *On the History of the Psycho-Analytic Movement* (Freud, 1914d) we find an account of his early ideas which seems hardly to square with the accounts he had given at the time. Here, twenty years later, he is contrasting the theory he had developed with that of Breuer. Breuer, he remarks, had "tried to explain the mental splitting in hysterical patients by the absence of communication between various mental states ... I had taken the matter less scientifically", continues Freud; "everywhere I seemed to discern motives and tendencies analogous to those of everyday life" (Freud, 1914d, p.11). The account of repression given as late as 1926 in his Encyclopaedia article continues in the same, almost rational, vein:

> There is a force in the mind which exercises the function of a censorship, and which excludes from consciousness and from any influence upon action all tendencies which displease it. Such tendencies are described as 'repressed'. They remain unconscious.
>
> (Freud, 1926f [1925], p.265)

In neither of these accounts are ideas of excessive excitation, of trauma or of primary repression to be found; instead, repression is represented as little more than an exaggeration of a desire to forget lapses and to avoid repeating them.

Nevertheless, throughout the middle period of his working life Freud seems to have been aware that there was more than one form of repression and it is therefore no surprise to find that in the final period from 1926 onwards he draws a clear distinction between the two:

"As I have shown elsewhere", he writes in *Inhibitions, Symptoms and Anxiety*:

> most of the repressions with which we have to deal in our therapeutic work are cases of after-pressure. They presuppose the operation of earlier, primal repressions which exert an attraction on the more recent situation. Far too little is known as yet about the background and preliminary stages of repression. There is a danger of over-estimating the part played in repression by the super-ego. We cannot at present say whether it is perhaps the emergence of primal repression and after-pressure. At any rate, the earliest outbreaks of anxiety, which are of a very intense kind, occur before the super-ego has become differentiated. It is highly probably that the

immediate precipitating causes of primal repressions are quantitative factors such as an excessive degree of excitation and the breaking through of the protective shield against stimuli.

(Freud, 1926d, p.94)

Here in the final sentence, trauma is rehabilitated. Thenceforward it reappears in each of the three main résumés he gives of his views: "The earliest and most fundamental repressions arise directly from traumatic factors, where the ego comes into contact with excessive libidinal demand" (*New Introductory Lectures*, Freud, 1933a, p.123). "Early trauma – Defence – Latency – Outbreak of the Neurosis – Partial Return of the repressed material: this was the formula we drew up for the development of the neuroses" (*Moses and Monotheism*, Freud, 1939a, p.129). "Instinctual demands from within operate as 'traumas' no less than excitations from the external world ... The helpless ego fends off these problems by attempts at flight (by repressions)" (Freud, 1940, p.61, *An Outline of Psycho-Analysis*).

There can be no doubt, therefore, that trauma has as central a place in Freud's later thinking about defence as it had had in the early phase. There is, however, one big difference in how he later conceives it. Up to 1920 trauma seems to be conceived as due solely to an excess of *external* stimulation: "We describe as 'traumatic' any excitations from outside which are powerful enough to break through the protective shield" (Freud, 1920g, p.29, *Beyond the Pleasure Principle*). In his later writings, as we have just seen, he sees it as arising from "excessive libidinal demand". This is a shift of viewpoint which, coupled with the concept of protective shield, can be used as the starting point for a fresh approach to the theory of defence.

The resulting formula "excessive instinctual demand, anxiety and trauma, defence" has, however, not proved a popular one. Probably because the second source of anxiety that Freud had described, and its related defences, is so much more readily understood, several formulations by leading analysts concentrate upon it almost to the exclusion of the traumatic. For example, the bulk of Fenichel's (1945) two chapters on defence discuss the difficulties and dangers to which satisfaction of the instincts are apt to lead in the external world and the resulting need to limit them. His phrase "the motives for defence are rooted in external influences" (Fenichel, 1945) sets the stage for his discourse. Only at one or two points, which will be noted later, does he depart from this viewpoint. Rapaport (1953) seems to go even further. In outlining the changes in Freud's concepts of the relation of defence to external reality he maintains that, from 1923 onwards, Freud held that "the ultimate motive (determiner) of defence is real danger, and the drive is defended against because if it were acted upon it would lead into a dangerous real situation. Thus defences against drives come to represent reality", Rapaport (1953, p.180).

As an account of Freud's later views it could hardly be more misleading. It is plain that Freud's concept of primary repression as resulting from an excessive strength of instinct that might damage the ego has proved puzzling. Nowhere, it seems, has it been taken as a starting point for theory construction. Usually after a brief reference, the discussion proceeds to easier terrain. Hartmann (1939) hazards that perhaps "the typical inability of the immature ego to provide gratification for drives is one of the reasons why instinctual drives are experienced as dangers", (Hartmann, 1939, p.104). Although Fenichel (1945) concurs, it is evident nonetheless that he regards such anxieties as little more than sensitisers:

> The infant, unable to attain satisfaction from his own efforts, necessarily often gets into traumatic situations, from which the first idea arises that instincts may be dangerous. The *more specific experiences show that instinctual acts may actually be dangerous.*
>
> (p.132, my italics)

A few pages later (p.142) he dismisses the idea that there may be "any innate primary anti-instinct forces", though whether or not he realises that in doing so he is also dismissing Freud's concept of primary repression is uncertain. From these two passages and an earlier one (p.51) there seems little doubt that it is the experience of the *results* of instinctual acts to which Fenichel attaches the greater weight.

The same seems true of Anna Freud (1936). Although she lists "dread of the strength of the instincts" as one of the "motives" for defence, she adds nothing to Freud's account. The paragraph in which she expresses her pessimism about the effects of analytic therapy for cases that show this feature,[10] moreover, suggests that she regards most of them as being psychotic. In her view, it seems, primary repression plays no great part in the neuroses or character disorders.

The position of Melanie Klein is, of course, very different. Like Freud, she recognises two distinct kinds of defensive process. The first she terms "splitting", the second "repression". Splitting, she holds, is the first and decisive process. On the form it takes turns the form taken later by repression, which, she believes, only assumes "a leading part among the defences" after the super-ego has become more integrated. "The extent to which splitting processes are resorted to ... vitally influences the use of repression at a later stage" (Klein et al., 1952, p.228).

---

10 [Bowlby notes:] "The only pathological states which fail to react favourably to analysis are those based on a defence prompted by the patient's dread of the strength of his instincts" (A. Freud, 1936, p.69).

How, we may ask, do Melanie Klein's concepts of splitting and repression relate respectively to Freud's concepts of primary and secondary repression? Melanie Klein herself does not discuss it,[11] nor, so far as I am aware, do her colleagues. Yet the more closely the two sets of ideas are examined the plainer it becomes that at a descriptive level there is much agreement. What Melanie Klein terms repression corresponds exactly with Freud's secondary repression. What Melanie Klein terms splitting seems almost certain to refer to the same phenomena as Freud explains by his concept primary repression. In each case the defence is held to have far-reaching effects on personality organization. The case for regarding the processes as essentially the same is, moreover, strengthened if we consider briefly two other defences that Freud described – secondary narcissism and splitting of the ego. Each, it will be argued, is closely related to what Freud terms primary repression and Melanie Klein splitting.

As regards secondary narcissism both Freud himself and Melanie Klein come near to making this equation. In describing the process of secondary narcissism Freud writes:

> The process which detaches the libido from its objects and blocks the way back to them again is closely allied to the process of repression, and is to be regarded as a counterpart of it .... [Moreover] the preliminary conditions giving rise to these [narcissistic] processes are almost identical, so far as we know at present, with those of repression.
>
> (Freud, 1916–1917, p.351)

From the context it seems clear that it is with what he was later to term primary, not secondary, repression that Freud is linking them. In a rather similar way, Melanie Klein links secondary narcissism to splitting, of which she believes it to be a result: "another typical feature of schizoid[12] object-relations," she writes, "is their narcissistic nature" (Klein et al., 1952, p.306). Thus primary repression, secondary narcissism and Kleinian splitting are seen to be close if not identical processes.

That the process termed by Freud splitting of the ego belongs also in the same family of defences as primary repression and secondary narcissism is evident also once the case material to which the terms are applied

---

11 [Bowlby notes:] In Melanie Klein's writings there appears to be only one brief reference to primary repression (1932, p.138). It precedes the elaboration of her ideas on splitting, which came ten years later.

12 [Bowlby notes:] Because they regard early splitting processes as those underlying schizophrenia both Melanie Klein (1952) and Fairbairn (1952) use the term "schizoid" as equivalent to splitting. Since I do not believe these processes are closely related to those giving rise to schizophrenia, I regard this usage as misleading.

is studied. (see Pathological mourning and childhood mourning, Bowlby, 1963). Since, however, the essential identity of this family of defences is a main theme of the rest of this paper, there is no need to discuss it further at this point.

Nevertheless, although at a descriptive level the process termed by Melanie Klein "splitting" is virtually identical with that termed by Freud "primary repression", in regard to their respective conceptions of how the process originates, at what time of life, and the function it serves, there is sharp divergence.

For Freud, as we have seen, primary repression is a process that is initiated by excess of libidinal demand and serves to protect the ego from disorganisation. It is especially liable to come into action between the ages of two and four years:

> All these traumata belong to early childhood.[13] ... The period between two and four years is the most important. How soon after birth this sensitiveness to traumata begins we are not able to state with any degree of certainty.
>
> (Freud, 1939a, pp.119–120)

Its effects, Freud holds, are usually perhaps always pathogenic. For Melanie Klein, on the other hand, splitting is a process adopted by the ego in order to defend itself against what she holds to be "the primordial anxiety ... the threat of annihilation by the death instinct within ...; it deflects to some extent that threat outwards" (Klein, 1957, p.22). "Splitting processes are resorted to in the first few months of life", she maintains (Klein et al., 1952, p.228), and they are indispensable for healthy development.

It will be apparent from my previous papers that as between these two conceptions of early defence my position will be closer to Freud's than to Melanie Klein's. Little evidence, it has been shown, has been presented for either of Melanie Klein's main hypotheses – that the primordial anxiety is a dread of annihilation and that the crucial period for psychological development is the first six months of life. I question also her hypothesis that splitting processes are indispensable to healthy development: it seems inherently unlikely.

The relation of defence to healthy control, or coping processes, has never been clarified. Like Melanie Klein, most analysts hold the view that there is no great difference between them. Rapaport (1953), for example, sees both as due to the activity of "counter-cathectic energy distributions", some of which, the defensive, "effectively prevent the execution of the

---

13 [Bowlby notes:] In this account Freud suggests "the period up to about five years"; [Editors' note: S. Freud (1939a).] ....in the *Outline* (p.51) it is "up to the age of six".

motivations against which they are directed" whilst "others, controlling ones, merely delay, modulate and channel motivations". Thus, "instead of a sharp dichotomy," he concludes, "we find a fluid transition". (Rapaport, 1953, p.193) In Hartmann's (1939), writings, also we find a rather similar viewpoint; for example, "defence processes may *simultaneously* serve both the control of instinctual drive and [also] adaptations to the external world", (Hartmann, 1939, p.50). Passages in some of Anna Freud's writings echo the same theme. For instance, in discussing the healthy development of young children she describes the way in which limitation is placed on the expression of "the wish to hurt people and later the wish to destroy objects ... They are usually first restricted, then suppressed, by commands and prohibitions; a little later they are repressed which means that they disappear from the child's consciousness" (Burlingham & Freud, 1942, p.30).

From the contexts in which these statements are made and from what we know of their views about defence in general, it seems clear that each of these statements is mainly concerned with secondary repression. And in regard to secondary repression Freud would probably have agreed. In regard to primary repression, on the other hand, Freud's position is very different. Not only did he hold that primary repression was the kind "with which we have to deal in our therapeutic work" (Freud, 1926d, p.94), but from his early description of it there can be no doubt that he conceived it as radically different in character from any process that can legitimately be referred to as healthy control.

In the light of this it comes as a surprise that Melanie Klein should hold not only that a moderate degree of (secondary) repression is necessary for healthy development, but that many other defences are so too. "Omnipotence, denial and idealization", she maintains, "enable the early ego to assert itself to a certain degree against its internal persecutors and against a slavish and perilous dependence upon its loved objects, and thus to make [possible] further advances in development" (Klein, 1940, p.130).

Splitting also is both necessary and desirable. Splitting, she claims, achieves two inter-related results. On the one hand, as we have seen, it is held to deflect the death instinct outwards and so is a means of preserving the ego. On the other, "it preserves the good object and later on enables the ego to synthesize the two aspects of it ... a certain amount of splitting is essential for integration" – a conclusion that Melanie Klein herself recognises to be paradoxical (Klein, 1957, pp.22–24).

The criterion for healthy control and therefore for mental health which I adopt is one already widely recognised: it is that of integration based on free communication and interaction between different parts of the mental apparatus (see Jahoda, 1958).[14] On this criterion, any process that leads to splits or to barriers to interaction is by definition pathological. So far from there being "a fluid transition" between them, defensive processes and controlling ones are seen as antithetical. It is a distinction well described by French (1938). "The ego is like a delicate electrical instrument that is completely thrown out of adjustment by too intense a current," he writes (1938). Its "normal function ... is its integrative function; defences are activated only when the integrative function has failed or is about to fail" (French, 1938, p.549).

Because processes of integrative control and those that lead to segregation are antithetical, only confusion can result from using the same term to denote both of them. In what follows, therefore, I shall confine the term "defence" to phenomena connected with splits and barriers – a usage that is closely in line with clinical practice. When I am referring to integrative control I shall use terms such as "controlling", "coping" and "regulating".

From the foregoing it seems plain that there are in psycho-analytic theory at least two distinct concepts of defence and that different schools of thought lay different emphasis upon them. Both concepts I believe to be valid. Since, however, it is my thesis that most of the pathology that follows loss is due to defences of the kind that Freud first described, later termed primary repression and always related to trauma, it is with this kind that I shall be dealing. The particular trauma with which we are concerned is, of course, that resulting from loss of mother.

Next we will turn to one of the most controversial aspects of the theory of defence, that of the twin problems of their causation and function.

Causation and function

It has long been recognised that how the causation and function of defence is conceived reflects the theory of anxiety that the analyst holds. The many who place weight on super-ego anxiety see defensive processes as guarding the ego from the dangerous consequences in the external world of the id's impetuous acts. Those who, like Melanie Klein, regard the primal danger as annihilation due to the effects of the death instinct within see defence as a means whereby the ego avoids being overtaken by a form of suicide. Those who, like Fairbairn, regard separation anxiety as central see defence

14 [Bowlby notes:] In her discussion of *Current Concepts of Positive Mental Health* Marie Jahoda (1958) treats "integration of the personality" as a major category of criterion. In reviewing the (American) literature she notes that this criterion is usually treated with emphasis on (a) balance of psychic forces; (b) a unifying (cognitive) outlook; or (c) resistance to stress. None of these, however, comprehend the concept of freedom of communication and interaction between motivational systems, a concept that in one version or another is prevalent in the British literature (e.g. Fairbairn, Melanie Klein, Winnicott).

as "a bipolar (aversive-appetitive) process".[15] Those who, like Freud, regard excessive internal excitation as endangering ego-organisation see defence as a means for preserving the integrity of the ego. Such diverse emphasis is well-known.

What perhaps is less well-known is that each theory of defence tends to reflect also a theory of motivation. Thus, if the model of motivation is exclusively an *avoidance* model, the accompanying theory of defence is likely also to be cast in an avoidance mould. Probably because this was in fact Freud's model of motivation, it was, too, his model of defence. Except for Fairbairn and Melanie Klein, almost all analysts have followed in the same tradition. It is not unexpected, therefore, that because by contrast I am adopting a different model of motivation – a model that regards avoidance as only one class of motivation and appetitive *behaviour* as another with different characteristics – the model of defence advanced here should differ substantially from traditional ones. On the other hand, because at many points my theory of anxiety resembles Freud's, there are also, as I have already indicated, many points at which my theory of defence resembles a principal one of his, that of primary repression. Let us begin with the divergences, many of which spring from differing theories of motivation.

It is well-known that very early in his psychological theorising Freud made what he later described as a "speculative assumption" (Freud, 1920g, p.7), namely that all motivation is initiated by unpleasurable tension that ends when tension is lowered:

> In the theory of psycho-analysis we have no hesitation in assuming that ... the course of [mental] events is invariably set in motion by an unpleasurable tension, and that it takes a direction such that its final outcome coincides with a lowering of that tension – that is, with an avoidance of unpleasure or a production of pleasure.

Thus run the opening sentences of *Beyond the Pleasure Principle* (Freud, 1920g, p.7); and the reality principle which he added does no more than enable the pleasure principle, or unpleasure principle as he originally termed it, to operate more effectively. Thus *all motivation is avoidance*.

The theory of motivation led him in turn to advance a theory of defence which is also an avoidance theory. From first to last he conceives of defences against internal stimuli as being modelled on the reactions by which we withdraw from painful stimuli that assail us in the external world. This view he argues in detail in the *Interpretation of Dreams* (Freud,

---

15 [Editors' note:] we have filled in a gap in the text here with the relevant quote from Fairbairn.

1900a). Whenever "the primitive apparatus is impinged upon by a perceptual stimulus which is a source of painful excitation", he remarks, the response is one of withdrawal. Furthermore, so far from there being any tendency to recall the source of pain, there will be a tendency "to drop the distressing memory-picture immediately, if anything happens to revive it ... The avoidance of the memory ... is [thus] no more than a repetition of the previous flight from the perception ...". From this he draws a conclusion that has influenced all further thinking: "This effortless and regular avoidance by the psychical process of the memory of anything that had once been distressing affords us the prototype and first example of *psychical repression*" (Freud, 1900a, p.600). A quarter of a century later he is still endorsing "the idea that a defence against an unwelcome *internal* process will be modelled upon the defence adopted against an *external* stimulus". Repression, he concludes, "is, fundamentally, an attempt at flight" (1926d, p.92, 153). He never revised it and only occasionally suggested an alternative.

A model of defence based on withdrawal and avoidance has the merit of simplicity and is indeed extremely plausible. Partly for that reason, no doubt, and partly because the avoidance theory of motivation can without too much difficulty be reconciled with a drive reduction theory of motivation (Dollard & Miller, 1950), the avoidance model of defence has been widely accepted.[16] Nevertheless, when we come to examine it, and the theory of motivation from which it stems, in the light of recent work on motivation theory and neuro-physiology, alternative and, I believe, more adequate models come to mind.

In the first place, despite the strenuous efforts of Hull (1943) and his followers to demonstrate the truth of the drive reduction theory of motivation, evidence of its inadequacy has steadily mounted. The attack has come from two sides – from psychology and from neurophysiology. From each source much data has accumulated that does not fit. Evidence has been well reviewed by both Peters (1958) and Deutsch (1960). Parallel with declining confidence in the drive reduction type of theory there has developed increasing support for an alternative type of theory, one that sees motivation as being of at least two different sorts, the aversive and the appetitive, each with its own characteristics. Today scientists as diverse as Harlow (1953), Hinde (1959), Nissen (1954), Schneirla (1959), Olds (1958),

---

16 [Bowlby notes:] Using as a model the drive reduction theory of motivation and postulating that anxiety acts as a drive, Dollard and Miller (1950) have elaborated a theory of this type. Repression, in their view, is closely related to conscious suppression and is based upon inhibition of thoughts and other responses that have become conditioned stimuli for anxiety. "Repression is the symptom of avoiding certain thoughts; it is reinforced by drive reduction in exactly the same way as the symptoms that have already been discussed."

and Magoun (1958) subscribe to this view. A very detailed model of appetitive behaviour, moreover, has been described by Deutsch (1953, 1960). Since it appears adequate to the data, it is claiming increasing interest.

There is no longer need, therefore, for the psycho-analyst to feel tied to an avoidance theory of motivation. On the contrary, he is in good company if he follows Fairbairn in adopting a bipolar (aversive-appetitive) theory. This gives him freedom to consider whether, perhaps, certain defences may not be more readily understood in terms of appetitive motivation than in terms of avoidance. The theory I am advancing springs naturally from combining Freud's formula "excessive instinctual demand, anxiety and trauma, defence" with a theory of motivation which regards appetitive behaviour as being distinct from and of at least equal importance to aversive.

Before leaving the avoidance model of defence it is necessary to draw attention to a peculiarity of it that seems to be responsible for an ambiguity that runs through much of the psycho-analytic literature. In the avoidance model the causes that initiate defences and the functions they serve are conceived as the mirror-images of one another. Anxiety and pain (or unpleasure) initiate them; the avoidance of anxiety and pain (or unpleasure) is their function. Largely perhaps as a result of this resemblance, in the literature on defence the discussion of causation is rarely kept distinct from that of function. Indeed, it seems that the need to keep the two issues distinct is not always appreciated, and for that reason it may be desirable to clarify them.

To the question "why in an animal is such and such a behavioural feature present?", ethologists point out, there are three altogether different kinds of answer possible. The first seeks to answer the question, what are the causal conditions that are necessary to evoke the behaviour; the second, what is the function, in terms of value for species survival that the behaviour serves; the third; by what steps in the course of evolution has the behavioural feature as we now see it come into being (Hinde, 1959).

Function is here conceived in terms of long-term biological advantage to the species and carries with it no suggestion of Aristotelian teleology as a causal principle (Pittendrigh, 1958). In this frame of reference, for example, we can conceive of photopositive behaviour usually being of advantage to a particular species of insect or bird without in any way suggesting that an insect or bird of that species is seeking the light because it wants to obtain the advantage in question. By the same reasoning we can conceive of processes of the kind that lead to defensive behaviour usually being of advantage to the species man without supposing that the individual in whom they occur initiates them because he wishes to obtain, or even knows about, that advantage. The position I shall take is that defensive processes come into action in certain conditions and that they do so without the individual having any more idea of their biological function than the ordinary man has of the function served by his temperature rising when he contracts an infection.

All too frequently these twin problems of the causation and function of defence are confounded. An example will illustrate the difficulty. In *An Autobiographical Study,* Freud (1925d) describes the origin of his basic ideas on defence:

> Everything that had been forgotten had in some way or other been distressing; it had been either alarming, or painful, or shameful by the standards of the subject's personality. It was impossible not to conclude that that was precisely why it had been forgotten.
>
> (Freud, 1925d, p.29)

Yet as an explanation this is unsatisfactory because ambiguous. One meaning is that alarm, pain and shame are conditions that are necessary for the initiation of processes of repression. Another is that, whatever the necessary causal conditions may be, the process of repression exists in humans in order to protect them from alarm, pain and shame of too high intensity. The first meaning refers to cause, the second to function but, because of the teleological form of the original statement, it is impossible to know which is intended.[17]

Before 1926, when he made his new approach to the problem, almost all Freud's statements about defence present the difficulties that arise from their being cast in a teleological form. Indeed these difficulties are inherent in the way that he first conceived of defence as a process akin to a wish to forget. In *Studies on Hysteria* (Freud, 1895d), in the very first passage in which the term repression is used, we read of how a patient who had "not reacted to a psychical trauma ... because it was a question of things the patient wished to forget and [had] therefore intentionally repressed from his conscious thought" (Freud, 1895d, p.10). This formulation is confirmed and amplified in the account he gives in *On the History of the Psycho-Analytic Movement* (Freud, 1914d), already referred to above where he attributes "psychical splitting" to "motives and tendencies analogous to those of everyday life" (Freud, 1914d, p.11).

It is this approach that was later developed into the concept of secondary repression and is the source of all those theories of defence in which some measure of foresight and purpose is attributed to an agency that

---

17 [Bowlby notes:] The same difficulty is present in Anna Freud's standard text, *The Ego and Mechanisms of Defence* (1936). Nowhere in this work is there discussion either of cause or function. Instead she speaks of "motives for the defence against instincts", and lists three: "object-anxiety", "super-ego anxiety", and "instinctual anxiety (namely dread of the strength of the instincts)". But whether these "motives" are to be regarded as the necessary conditions for evoking defence or as the functions that they serve is never stated.

effects the defence. As a rule the ego is credited both with some awareness that a painful or dangerous situation is impending and also with a capacity for planned action to meet it. Not until *Inhibitions, Symptoms and Anxiety* (Freud, 1926d), we have seen, was Freud able effectively to formulate his traumatic theory of defence: he there postulates that certain processes protect the ego from becoming disorganised by exposure to excessive strength of instinct. Not only is this type of theory more in keeping with the empirical data but it avoids also the problems of teleology: as a result it does not confound causation and function.

As regards causal conditions Freud advances the view that "it is highly probable that the immediate precipitating causes of primal repressions are quantitative factors such as an excessive degree of excitation", (Freud, 1926d, p.94) or, as he puts it elsewhere, "excessive libidinal demand" (1933a, p.123). Their function, he holds, is to prevent the dynamic organisation characteristic of the ego from being destroyed (Freud, 1949, p.70). Here is a clear distinction between cause and function; the cause is the magnitude of excitation, the function that of preserving ego-organisation.

It is of interest that it was from this standpoint that Freud approached the problem of defences that follow loss. It is from this standpoint also that my approach is made.

Defensive processes evoked by loss

Segregation of psychic systems

Study of the clinical data shows that in young children during a period of separation from their mothers and in older persons in states of pathological mourning two independent psychic systems co-exist. One system is oriented towards the lost object, longs for it, strives to recover it, and reproaches it for its desertion; the other system recognises its loss and organises behaviour on that basis. Of the two systems it is usual for the one that recognises loss to be more dominant than the other. The system that remains oriented towards the lost object varies in state from case to case. In some it is fully conscious and even reasonably well adapted to reality, as in the case of Mrs. Q, who after her father's sudden death in hospital made secret plans to recover him and welcome him home again. In others it is completely unconscious and little adapted, as in the case of Helene Deutsch's patient who, after his mother's death when he was a child, had a fantasy that a big dog would visit him.[18] No matter what

18 [Bowlby notes:] These and other cases referred to are reported in an earlier paper, "Pathological Mourning and Childhood Mourning". [Editors' note:] J. Bowlby (1963).

the particular state of the two systems may be, however, all these cases have one feature in common: the two co-existing systems are in some way divided one from another.

A number of terms have been employed to denote the process or processes that do the dividing – repression, denial, splitting. None has been used consistently, however, and it cannot be taken for granted that primary and secondary repression are identical.

No doubt because it is so much more readily understood, much of the theorising about defences that follow loss is in terms of secondary repression. Many analysts have concentrated so much on the role of guilt that the anxiety and painfulness of *yearning* have often been neglected. Whilst recognizing that guilt and therefore secondary repression play a part, it is my thesis that they are not the main factors. On the contrary, loss, it seems to me, is better conceived as a traumatic situation of the kind that evokes a more primitive type of defence – the kind termed by Freud primary repression and by Fairbairn and Melanie Klein splitting. Secondary repression, therefore, will concern us no further.

This leaves primary repression, denial and splits in the ego, the last the term used by Freud in his later work to describe cases such as Mrs. Q in which both systems are conscious. What, it may be asked, do each of these three terms denote? Do they denote three different processes or do they, perhaps, denote variants of only one? Let us examine the cases to which each term is applied. In doing so it is useful to proceed in two stages: first to consider the relatedness of primary repression to ego-splits and secondly its relatedness to denial.

Helene Deutsch's patient with the dog fantasy provides a good example of repression. This man's yearning for his lost mother seems to have become totally unconscious and almost inert; yet we know that in the years immediately after his loss it was sufficiently active to have given rise to the fantasy. Another case in which repression set in was the boy in the Hampstead Nurseries who at first enacted dramatically how his mother would come for him and dress him in coat and pixie hat but in whom the yearning later became unconscious and the acting an apparently meaningless ritual. Though it would be possible to regard each case as one of secondary repression, there appears to be no evidence for doing so; it is therefore just as plausible to regard them, as I do, as cases of primary repression. In each case the term repression is used because there is evidence of a psychic system with its accompanying affects and fantasies that is not only alien to the patient's conscious self with which we are in communication but which is kept shut off from and unknown to it by some powerful force. It is indeed to this force that the term repression applies.

The dynamic condition of patients in whom a split in the ego is said to be present, for example Mrs. Q, is, however, little different. Once again there is evidence of a psychic system with its accompanying affects and fantasies that is alien to the one with which we as analysts are in communication; once again there is evidence that it is kept shut off from it by some powerful force. The only difference seems to be that, whereas in the case of repression the alien system is to a greater or less degree unconscious, in the case of ego-split it is fully conscious. This is a difference that ceases to be of great consequence, however, once Freud's first model of the mental apparatus has been discarded and consciousness is no longer regarded as a basic criterion for distinguishing systems.

The question arises, therefore, in what way does the process, active in cases of primary repression, differ from the process active in cases of ego-split. Are they really so very different? Or are the processes essentially the same and only the outcomes a little different? The principle of parsimony in theory construction, it seems to me, requires us to postulate that, unless shown otherwise, the processes occurring in the two kinds of case are best regarded as variants of one and the same process. This is in accord with clinical experience. In clinical practice, as Freud himself points out, "it is not always easy to decide in the individual case with which of the two possibilities one is dealing" (1940a [1938], p.204).

Essentially the same conclusion is reached when the relatedness of denial to primary repression is examined. In Lewin's phrase, the distinction that Freud draws is that "denial disclaims the external world as repression disclaims the instincts" (Lewin, 1950, p.53). The validity of this distinction, however, turns on regarding instincts and external world as psychologically separate from one another. Empirically I doubt whether this is ever so. Each psychic system and its accompanying affect and fantasy, whether conscious or unconscious, is habitually directed towards some object believed to exist in the external world; whilst objects of the external world are probably only of psychological reality when they are taken as the objects of a psychic system and its affect and fantasies. Where in a personality there are contrary and independent psychic systems present each of the systems is found to be made up of motivational, affective, and cognitive components intrinsically linked. Thus, for example, when loss has been sustained the urge to recover the object, the longing and the anger, and also the picture of the lost object as still desirable and recoverable all belong to one system and this may be segregated from another system, all the components of which, motivational, affective and cognitive, take for granted the fact of loss. To use one term for the process that segregates different motives and affects from each other and another for the process that segregates different cognitive pictures of the object from each other is misleading. All components, it is clear, are potentially subject to the same segregating process, and a single generic term is required to denote it.

Both because each of the terms at present in use is associated with a theoretical model that, as I shall show later, has serious shortcomings and also because they have been used in such a diversity of ways, it is doubtful whether any one of them is eligible for general duty. The term "denial" has a cognitive flavour and has been applied by Freud specifically to the cognitive component. The term "split", although originally used by Freud (1914d) as a general descriptive term, was later employed by him in a way that presupposes the ego–id dichotomy. Later still, moreover, it has been employed by Fairbairn and Melanie Klein (Klein et al., 1952) in a way quite different again. The term "repression" has always been used to denote processes that keep something unconscious, and is therefore ill-suited to denote one that can also segregate two systems both of which are conscious. Over the years also it has come to be closely linked to the id–ego–super-ego model. To avoid these associations, therefore, and also to relate the concept I am using to that of integration, I am introducing the generic term "to segregate" and "segregating process"; they denote any process that creates barriers to communication and interaction between one psychic system and another.[19] Repression, primary or secondary, I shall confine to the common though nonetheless special cases in which one system is dominant and conscious and the other subordinate and unconscious: in this context primary and secondary repression denote two particular sorts of segregating process. In a similar way other additional terms are required for the many other particular sorts of segregating process.[20]

It is not, however, my intention to discuss particular sorts of process; before varieties can be defined and named it is wise to clarify the nature of the segregating process itself, that process which creates barriers to communication and interaction between one part of the apparatus and another. For it is these barriers to communication and interaction which are the essence of resistance as we meet it clinically; and it is the analyst's experience of resistance, as Freud frequently emphasised, that is the starting point for all theorising about defence. Concentration of attention on the co-existence of contrary and independent systems, and on the processes that segregate them which are encountered as resistance, is the point from which Freud's own theorising about defensive processes began, and it is to this point, I believe, that in our examination of defences that follow loss we are wise to return.

At a descriptive level, the state of a personality in which, following loss, defensive processes have been evoked is that two independent and segregated psychic systems have been brought into being. Depending on the case, each system is in greater or less degree reality oriented, and in greater

---

19 [Editors' note:] At this point in the manuscript, Bowlby makes a handwritten note: "dissociation".

20 [Bowlby notes:] Examples might be isolating and undoing, processes which Freud referred to as "variations of repression" (Freud, 1926d, p.119).

or less degree conscious. To these varying degrees of orientation to reality and of consciousness, the array of varying clinical pictures that are to be traced to pathological mourning is to be attributed.

Were the task I set myself to be an explanation of how and why these clinical conditions differ from one another it would of course be necessary to explore both the processes that lead to variation in orientation to reality and consciousness and also the conditions that promote each type of variation. My task, however, is a different and prior one. It is to understand, so far as possible, first, the nature of the processes that segregate these co-existent systems, secondly, the conditions that are necessary to set these processes in action, and, thirdly, the functions in the life of the individual or species that they serve; in a word their nature, causation and function.

Nature of process and causation

Following loss, we have seen, segregating processes of a pathological kind are apt to be evoked. To understand what causes them requires, first, an hypothesis about their nature. In *Inhibitions, Symptoms and Anxiety* Freud (1926d) threw out a suggestion on which I shall build.

In a discussion of some defensive processes that he regards as "variants of repression" Freud likens one of them, isolation, to "the normal phenomenon of concentration. Even a normal person uses concentration to keep away not only what is irrelevant or unimportant, but, above all, what is unsuitable because it is contradictory.... Thus, in the normal course of things, the ego has a great deal of isolating work to do" (Freud, 1926d, p.121). "In carrying out our analytic techniques", he continues, we "train it to relinquish that function" (Freud, 1926d, p.121).

In this passage the process of repression is regarded as a special example of the way attention is narrowed during concentration, and the process of overcoming resistance during therapy with that of broadening it again.

Far more is now known about these processes of selective exclusion than was known in Freud's day. Five sets of data are of special interest:

(i) processes of selective exclusion of input and output are an integral part of the action of the Central Nervous System (CNS) and so of mental organisation,

(ii) these processes increase the degree of exclusion as motivation is raised,

(iii) when an organism remains for a period in a state of unterminated high motivation the processes, already intensely active, often become rigid, and so irreversible,

(iv) the mechanism responsible for these processes operates erratically and inefficiently when the CNS is immature during the early years of life, and, it seems probable, is at that time especially sensitive to derangement,

(v) processes responsible for selective exclusion are closely related to, and perhaps in some respects identical with, processes governing consciousness and unconsciousness.

These data, it will be argued, support the following hypothesis regarding the nature of the defences that follow loss of mother in early childhood.

The pathological segregating processes that follow loss in early childhood are the form taken by normal processes of selective exclusion when they have become fixated in a deranged condition. Then derangement occurs because of their inherent sensitivity at this time of life and because loss leads them to be intensely active over a long period due to the unterminated high motivation that follows it.

Evidence in regard to each of the five sets of data will be reviewed.

***

Set (i) Evidence in regard to the mode of action of processes of selective exclusion, affecting both information and motor patterns, is substantial. It has long been plain that *every motor act* is determined by the integration in a unique pattern of a particular selection of information. This term I am using to cover receptor events stemming from three sources; those that derive from the environment (distal events), those that derive from the organism's body (proximal events), and those that derive from past experience stored in the CNS itself. Little is known as yet of how all this information is integrated, but recent work in neurophysiology and psychology has revolutionised our understanding of how it is selected.[21]

Selection of *information* is centrally regulated and as active a process as choosing a hat. Evidence comes from both psychology and neurophysiology (see Magoun, 1958; Livingston, 1959 for excellent reviews). Since the neurophysiological evidence is the more conclusive, we will consider it first.

For stimuli derived from the environment central selection and regulation is well demonstrated by experiments such as that of Hernandez-Peon and Hagbarth (1955a, 1955b). The transmission of auditory stimuli in the CNS of a healthy active cat was studied by means of electrodes placed in the cochlear nucleus. A metronome provided a rhythmic clicking noise. So long as the cat was undistracted and drowsy, regular electrical responses in

---

21 [Bowlby notes:] Pribram (1960, p.3) defines stimuli as "centrally regulated receptor events" thereby including both "distal" events deriving from the environment and "proximal" events deriving from the organism. (He reserves the term "input" for those receptor events which can be shown to be systematically related to an ensemble of environmental events".). Although according to Pribram's definition information deriving from past experience stored in the CNS (e.g. cognitive maps) could be termed stimuli, such an extension of the term would be confusing. My term "information" includes both kinds of stimuli and also information stored in the CNS.

the nucleus showed the rhythmic clicks from the metronome were being registered there. As soon as the cat was distracted, however, either by the sight of mice or by the smell of fish, the electrical responses ceased. Thus afferent impulses representing the uninteresting clicks from the metronome were being suppressed at some point peripheral to the nucleus while stimuli of greater interest were admitted. Once the sight of mice or smell of fish had been removed and the cat had resumed its drowsy state a resumption of the regular electrical responses in the nucleus showed that the suppression had ceased.

Thus, in regard to exteroceptive stimuli, the CNS performs a task of selective exclusion. Certain stimuli are accepted, others rejected. To perform it, the CNS is equipped with efferent neurons running from the higher centres either to the sense organs themselves (Kuffler, 1953) or else to a relay station between the sense organ and the centre. By these means stimuli are excluded at the periphery on instructions from the centre.

Psychological evidence for a comparable type of exclusion stems from experiments on human perception. Postman et al. (1948) have demonstrated that, when words are shown tachistoscopically, those that are related to a subject's preferred value categories are recognised more readily than those belonging to his low value categories. Not only this, however, but evidence suggests that "value orientation... also erects barriers against percepts and hypotheses incongruent with or threatening to the individual's values": the evidence they cite is that pre-solution responses to low-value words tend to be either nonsense or else contra-valuant. This suggests that at an unconscious level the subject first recognises the unwelcome word and then suppresses or distorts the message. "We suggest," conclude the authors, "that a defence mechanism similar to repression operates in perceptual behaviour" (Postman et al., 1948, p.152). If this is so it is presumably a process similar in kind to the one which excludes an uninteresting auditory click, though probably acting at a higher level of reception.[22]

---

22 [Bowlby notes:] Erikson (1954) reports similar findings but, subsequently (Eriksen & Browne, 1956), has questioned the plausibility of the Postman et al's (1948) hypothesis of perceptual defence on the grounds that it assumes "unconscious perceiving". The authors argue that instead perceptual defence can better be described in terms of the principles of behaviour theory derived from avoidance conditioning and punishment, along the lines of Dollard and Miller's (1950) theory of repression. This reluctance to accept as plausible a theory which assumes "unconscious perception" is in striking contrast to the readiness with which neurophysiologists nowadays postulate it: "Briefly" writes Livingston (1959), "this sensory control mechanism appears to provide the perceptual processes with an active organising principle, including an element of purpose, which tends to select and modify sensory messages within the earliest stages of their trajectory... A mechanism operating in this way requires that incoming signals be identified and given significance... The attachment of value to such identified signals could presumably come about quite naturally through the activation, *pari passu*, of certain portions of the brain's primary reinforcement systems" (Livingston, 1959).

There is evidence also that similar mechanisms are present to exercise selective exclusion of proprioceptive stimuli. For example, whether or not pain is experienced turns on much else beside the state of the damaged limb or organ. As every athlete knows, any situation that attracts intense, prolonged attention may diminish or abolish pain perception. It seems probable that, in the far from simple process of afferent transmission of electrical impulses evoked by painful stimuli, there are relay stations at which the impulses can be suppressed before they reach the centre. Much work is now in progress on the means whereby suppression is achieved and on the routes taken by the corticofugal pathways that carry the suppressing instructions (Melzack et al., 1958).

Thus as regards exteroceptive and proprioceptive stimuli there is good evidence both from neurophysiology and psychology that a process of central regulation leads to some stimuli being accepted and others rejected, and that such selective exclusion is proceeding every minute of our lives. As regards information from the third source, that deriving from past experience stored in the CNS, though there is as yet no evidence of selective exclusion from neurophysiology, there is much from psychology. An example is the way in which in the normal process of concentration irrelevant thoughts and considerations are excluded in favour of those that are relevant (Bartlett, 1932). A more dramatic one is what happens during hypnosis. As Barber (1958) has argued, hypnosis can best be understood as an interpersonal relationship characterised by a number of special processes in the subject. A principal one is the subject's exclusion of all stimuli (exteroceptive and proprioceptive) excepting only "the words of the hypnotist and those aspects of his self and his surroundings to which the hypnotist specifically directs his attention", (Barber, 1958, p.118). A second is his exclusion of all modes of interpreting his relation to his environment excepting those which are in accordance with the hypnotist's definitions. Thus, if a friend is defined by the hypnotist as an enemy he will be attacked; if a wallet is defined by the hypnotist as the subject's own it will be stolen. A single conceptual schema, that provided by the hypnotist, determines action, because all alternative schemas are excluded.

Selective exclusion, therefore, affects information from each of the three main sources and takes place at many different levels. So deeply are the neurophysiologists impressed by their findings, indeed, that they have concluded: "It would appear that the central nervous system has as precise control over its input as over its output" (Livingston & Hernandez-Peon, 1955, p.280).

The selective exclusion of *organised motor patterns* is of equal relevance and, once again, the work of the neurophysiologists is of interest. In the course of ontogeny complex motor patterns come to be organised as autonomous units. Thenceforward they persist in active or latent form. Even when they have become dysfunctional they remain present and are only prevented from being troublesome by an active process of exclusion.

An example is given by Weiss and Sperry,[23] who describe experiments on polio patients in whom the attachment of muscle tendons is shifted to enable them to use an intact muscle in place of one that is paralysed. The attached muscle tendon may now have to move a joint in a direction opposite to the one in which it normally moves it. Though with practice the patient can learn to use the muscle in its new role, not infrequently the muscle relapses into its old one which, thanks to the changed attachment, makes for chaotic movement.

"It must be concluded, therefore", writes Weiss (1950), "that there has been no remodelling of the old [pre-operative] pattern itself, but that a wholly new pattern... had been set up on a higher level to substitute functionally for the inadequate [old] one. The latter remained latent but retained its integrity and reappeared periodically whenever the higher replacement went into recess," as for example when the patient was tired.

Elsewhere Weiss protests vigorously against a picture of the CNS, held by some psychologists, which sees it as a monotonic network of units which undergo recombination every time a new act is substituted for an old one.

Actually the work of the experimental psychologists themselves strongly supports Weiss's view. Every learned motor response that has been "extinguished" has a tendency to reappear after an interval, showing that in the intervening period it remains an organised whole. It is as though every fire that was thought extinguished smouldered on to blaze afresh. A fire brigade that described such fires as "extinguished" would rightly be criticised. It is unfortunate that in psychology this term has become so established that it will be difficult to replace. For it obscures the crucial fact that motor patterns, however inappropriate and dysfunctional they may be, tend to persist and are only rendered inoperative by active processes of exclusion.[24]

Evidence of the constant activity of processes of selective exclusion, both in regard to information and to motor output, is therefore substantial. Evidence that something similar occurs with those larger behavioural units I am terming psychic systems derives from everyday life: a young man in love will have difficulty in attending to his work. Here both information and motor output suffers from selective exclusion. The neurophysiologist is not surprised by the existence of such a complex unit: "there is really no physiological boundary between central sensory and motor mechanisms. Each central pattern for the initiation of

---

23 [Editors' note:] Bowlby cites Weiss and Sperry without a date. No joint reference was found but the intended reference is likely to be Weiss and Brown (1941) and/or R. W. Sperry (1945).

24 [Bowlby notes]: A paragraph here is required on Harlow's theory of learning. [Editors' notes:] For example H. F. Harlow (1936 & Harlow, 1952).

movement has its neuronal repercussions upon central sensory patterns, and each performed movement introduces alterations in sensory input patterns" (Livingston, 1959).

There can be no doubt, therefore, that selective exclusion is an integral and ubiquitous part of the action of the CNS. That the segregating processes characteristic of pathological defence may be special cases of it was, as we have seen, adumbrated by Freud in 1926, though he never elaborated the idea. It happens that a few years earlier in *Beyond the Pleasure Principle* (Freud, 1920g) he had made a related suggestion, that of "a protective shield against stimuli" (Freud, 1920g, pp.27–31). It is, however, appreciably further from the present hypothesis than his later one, since, in describing it, he postulates that the shield is operative only against *external* stimuli and also that its function is to defend the organism against lethal energies. Indeed, in contrast to the hypothesis advanced here, he lays much emphasis then and later on the idea that the shield is inoperative against stimuli of internal origin; "the protective shield exists only in regard to external stimuli, not in regard to internal instinctual demands" (Freud, 1926d, p.94). It is this, indeed, that he regards as creating the great problem for ego organisation. Yet, even with these provisos, a conclusion he reached in 1920 has about it a modern ring: "Protection against stimuli is an almost more important function for the living organism than reception of stimuli" (Freud, 1920g, p.27).

In the later passage, as we have seen, Freud's formulation is virtually identical with that proposed here; and in it he identifies the therapeutic process of overcoming resistance with that of relinquishing selective exclusion. As every analyst knows, usually it is not easy.

Ease or difficulty of reversal is, indeed, the criterion that distinguishes health from pathology. Selective exclusion, both of information and of motor output, proceeds every moment of our lives. What characterises a pathological condition is that exclusion acts in such a way that it creates not only the usual temporary barrier but a permanent one. Thereby psychic systems are segregated from one another as though by an iron curtain.

How and in what circumstances, we may ask, is this apt to occur? Much evidence, deriving from the second and third of our five main sets of data, suggests that a major cause is a state of high motivation that remains unterminated over a period, such as occurs following loss. Since the evidence is of two kinds, the argument is in two steps. The first kind shows the increase in selective exclusion caused by high motivation; the second kind that responses adopted in conditions of high motivation tend to become stereotyped and fixated.

***

Set (ii) It is now well-established that within certain limits the higher the motivation the greater the selective exclusion both of information and of motor output. An early experiment was by Bahrick et al. (1952).

They gave two groups of subjects a main task (tracking a pursuit meter); one group was told it was only a practice run whilst the other was encouraged to try hard by the prospect of earning a bonus, rising with performance. During the course of doing this task, and without previous warning, what amounted to a second task was introduced: peripheral lights were switched on in a certain order, and later the subjects were asked to describe this order. Results showed that, whilst the high incentive increased performance on the main task, performance on the peripheral task was impaired. This means that as incentive increases subjects show a higher degree of selective attention for those parts of the perceptual field they judge important, with a concomitant tendency to exclude from attention parts they judge unimportant.[25] Rats exhibit the same tendency (Bruner et al., 1955). Furthermore, whereas in conditions of moderate motivation the individual will vary his attempts to solve the problem facing him, abandoning courses that prove useless and trying others, in conditions of high motivation he is apt to stick rigidly to a single course of action despite its leading only to failure. In rats a reduction of trial and error movements is observed; in humans a tendency to stick to a single approach not noticing that the plan adopted fails to meet the requirements of the problem.

An amusing illustration is recounted by Bruner (personal communication). The subject is presented with a pithball at the bottom of a cylindrical jar, a wire, pincers and a flask of ginger ale, and is instructed to recover the pithball without moving the jar. Both wire and pincers are found too short. Although pouring the ginger ale into the flask to float the pithball to the top provides an easy solution, subjects who are confronted with the task when thirsty are less likely than otherwise to hit on it: thirst fixates them too strongly on another usage for the ginger ale.[26] In a rather similar way chimpanzees, well used to employing a stick to help obtain food placed out of reach, when unduly hungry limit themselves fruitlessly to reaching with their arm alone (Birch, 1945).

Such experiments demonstrate clearly that under conditions of high motivation performance is based on the integration of a much reduced quantity of information, both that obtained from external (perceptual) sources and also that drawn from internal (stored) sources. The repertoire of available motor patterns is restricted also.

***

25 [Bowlby notes:] Bahrick et al. (1954) reports a further experiment, also with humans, with the same results.
26 [Bowlby notes:] See also the experiment reported by M. D. S. Ainsworth, & L. H. Ainsworth (1958).

Set (iii) Our third set of data, that relating to the tendency for patterns of performance to become fixated in conditions of unterminated high motivation, is to be found in the extensive literature on responses to situations of psychosocial stress. For, as Scott (1949)[27] has pointed out, "a stress situation ... may be defined as one in which adjustment is difficult or impossible but in which motivation is very strong".

Initially, as we have seen, in conditions of high motivation there is much restriction both of information and of action patterns. Next, there follows a partial breakdown in this process of exclusion: as regards information, it is shown by increasing distractibility; as regards behaviour, which is tightly organised during the initial phase, it is shown by the appearance of other, often primitive, responses, which at first interfere with it and may later replace it altogether.[28] Finally, if unterminated high motivation persists, the state that the organism reaches, as regards the exclusion both of information and of motor repertoire, becomes relatively permanent.

Many examples of behaviour becoming fixated in such conditions are given in the studies of experimental neuroses by Liddell[29] (1956) and Massermann[30] (1943). An example from the behaviour of birds reported by Hinde (1960) is of particular interest because it occurs in a situation in which an object indispensable for normal behaviour is missing. When a canary in its first spring is deprived of nest-building material, its urge to build is such that it will develop alternative building behaviour, e.g. using its own feathers, which is ineffectual and maladaptive. After being adopted in the chaffinches' first season and even when adequate material is provided in later ones, it persists. For the remainder of its life its nest-building behaviour is maladaptive.

That the motor responses adopted in such conditions of stress tend to become fixated and so to lead to pathological behaviour is now fairly well-known (Hinde, 1960; Schaffer, 1954; Scott, 1957). What perhaps is less clearly recognised is that the underlying mechanism of selective exclusion itself becomes deranged. Instead of being sensitive, efficient and reversible, it becomes stuck in a condition that is at once restrictive, erratic and rigid [note in margin: contradiction]. Not only are information and motor responses relevant to any one goal narrowly restricted but information and motor responses relevant to some other and perhaps incompatible goal may be allowed through. It is as though an enquiry

27 [Editors' note:] This might be J. P. Scott (1949).
28 [Bowlby notes:] It seems likely that the tendency to "unrepression" during exposure to psychological stress reported by Janis (1958) is an effect of this breakdown of selective exclusion.
29 [Editors' note:] This may be a reference to H. S. Liddell (1956).
30 [Editors' note:] Possibly J.H. Masserman (1943).

clerk, when asked about trains to Cornwall, gave information endlessly about the night express to Plymouth with occasional intrusions about a plane to Rome.

A model of this kind to explain the segregating processes that follow loss and initiate pathology is not original. In addition to the ideas regarding isolation mooted by Freud, Tolman (1948) has sketched a model identical with it. In a famous paper on *Cognitive Maps in Rats and Men,* Tolman reaches the conclusion that "some, at least, of the so-called 'psychological mechanisms'... can be interpreted as narrowings of our cognitive maps due to too strong motivations or to too intense frustrations". Nevertheless, although he discusses fixation and regression and also displacement (redirection) in these terms, he does not apply them to the problem of repression. Nor does he relate them to the special characteristics of processes of selective exclusion found in the immature – our fourth main set of data.

***

Set (iv) There is evidence that, in comparison with the adult, processes of selective exclusion in the child operate both inefficiently and erratically, and that, in general, the younger the child the more inefficient and the more erratic they are.

The child's inefficient selection of external stimuli is shown by his tendency to pay *excessive* attention to irrelevant stimuli and too little to relevant ones. Because so easily distracted his span of attention is short: conversely, when visual or auditory stimuli are called to his attention, he is extremely slow to register them. Moreover, as experiments reported by Russian psychologists show, he has much difficulty in preventing stimuli he knows to be irrelevant from influencing his motor responses. An example is an experiment reported by Paramonova (1956).[31] Three-year-olds were taught to press a key in response to a light signal of a particular colour. Despite understanding clearly that they were not to respond when lights of other colours were shown, they habitually did so. Many years earlier Luria (1932) drew attention to the difficulty that children of under seven years have in moving their finger selectively towards a point indicated by the experimenter. When one of five cards spread before him is indicated, instead of touching it the young child usually moves his finger impulsively towards the card nearest him. Luria also drew attention to the great difficulty young children have in imposing any delay on their responses.

Their difficulty in imposing delay was demonstrated again by an experiment of Lambercier and Rey (1935).[32] In the presence of a reward that is visible but out of reach, children aged four to five years are so fixated on direct attempts to reach it that they are unable to explore alternative ways

31 [Bowlby notes:] Both these experiments are quoted by Vince (1961).
32 [Bowlby notes:] See previous footnote above.

of obtaining it. In other words, they behave habitually much as do an adult human or a chimpanzee when in a condition of high motivation.

This difficulty in imposing delay is consistent with and helps to explain Miller's conclusion that the younger the child the more is he likely to resort to defences of denial and fantasy. Miller et al. (1960) presented children of different ages with a story-completion test in which the hero is prevented from reaching his goal (either because an adult lets him down or accidentally frustrates him). When asked to complete such stories the younger the child the more likely is he to maintain that, despite all, the hero nonetheless attains his objective. For example, nearly half the answers of children even as old as seven to nine years are of this kind. Thus, the young child tries to proceed headlong to his goal, unable to take into account new and inconvenient information.

Immatures of lower species show the same characteristics. For example, in her study of learning in birds Vince (1958) found that juveniles were ill-equipped compared to adults in their capacity to restrict useless responses. She points out further (1961), that the findings of Thompson and Heron (1954) with dogs suggests that this reduced ability of immatures is attributable, partly at least, to their experience. Adult dogs which have been reared in restricted conditions are virtually incapable of the delayed reactions typical of an ordinary adult; for example, like young children, they persist in running straight for food even when repeatedly obstructed by wire-netting.

Another result of inefficiency in the processes of selective exclusion in the immature, and one that may be of great consequence for psychopathology, is the increased tendency of young children compared to adults, to return to an uncompleted task. This was first reported by Zeigarnik (1927).[33]

Here again similarities with the findings of neurophysiology may be relevant. Motor patterns, it has been emphasised, have a way of persisting at a latent level and of becoming manifest after an interval even when dysfunctional. Patterns specially prone to this, Weiss (1955) remarks, are those in which genetic influences play a preponderant part. If we are right in supposing the response systems underlying the child's tie to his mother to be in this category, their persisting latent activity following loss of object is exactly what would be expected.

***

Set (v) Our fifth and last set of data concerns the relatedness of processes of selective exclusion to those governing consciousness. Although in his theory of defence Freud abandoned the distinction consciousness–unconsciousness as a fundamental criterion, it is nevertheless obvious that a main effect of defensive processes is to render unconscious much

---

33 [Bowlby notes:] Literature still to be studied.

motivation, affect and fantasy that would otherwise be conscious. It would be strange and unsatisfactory, therefore, were it difficult to relate a theory of defensive process to a theory of processes governing consciousness. It is believed that the theory advanced here presents no such difficulty. Evidence from both neuroanatomy and introspection suggests, indeed, that the processes are closely related to one another.

The cerebral system mainly responsible for selective exclusion and integration is the same as that responsible for consciousness and unconsciousness: it is the brainstem reticular formation. Work of the past decade suggests, however, that, although both processes are mediated by a single system, they may be mediated by rather different parts of it (Magoun, 1958). An upper, or thalamic, component is thought to be mainly responsible for processes of selective exclusion and integration in the conscious animal, whilst a lower brain-stem component, less sensitive to differences between stimuli, produces long-lasting changes in reactivity, such as that between sleep and wake. Nevertheless, although some differentiation of function seems probable, the two components of the system are closely related anatomically. It seems likely, therefore, that the functions they serve are closely related also.

Evidence from introspection points to the same conclusion. Whereas some degree of selective exclusion, as for example, during intense concentration, seems to heighten consciousness, when increased beyond a certain point consciousness is lowered. This is evident in sleep and hypnosis; it is evident also in conditions of unterminated high motivation. Both rage and love are apt to make us blind. Loss of temper, indeed, can at times amount almost to loss of consciousness.

Conversely, consciousness seems to be heightened when selective exclusion is reduced so that more information and a greater variety of possible actions are together permitted integration. Cobb (1952) has suggested that "it is the integration itself, the relationship of one functioning part to another, which is mind and which causes the phenomenon of consciousness"; and Fessard (1954) has accordingly proposed that consciousness be termed an "Experienced Integration". "Consciousness," he writes, "seems to be linked with the preparation of action rather than with action actually taking place... it is more often linked with deferred action".

If this analysis is correct, consciousness tends to *vary inversely* with the activity of the normal processes selective exclusion. From this it follows that, when the activity of these processes is not only increased beyond a certain point but remains fixated in that condition, motivation, affect and fantasy that would otherwise be pre-conscious (mainly available for consciousness) is rendered unconscious. This is a conclusion in keeping with the theory of defence advanced.

This completes our review of the five main sets of data. The theory proposed – regarding the nature of pathological defensive processes and of the causal conditions that evoke them is claimed to have a number of merits. It fits the data regarding responses to loss; it is concordant with knowledge, both neurophysiological and psychological, of healthy processes of selective exclusion and integration; it is supported by evidence both of the effects on these processes of stressors and of their state of functioning in the immature; and it can be related plausibly with a theory of processes responsible for consciousness. Finally, it can be brought into satisfactory relationship with a theory of anxiety which itself fits the data on responses to loss.

In an earlier paper (Bowlby, 1960) I advanced the hypothesis that primary anxiety is experienced whenever and instinctual response system is activated but not terminated and, further, that the more intensely the system is activated the more intense the anxiety. In this one I have suggested that pathological defence processes are evoked when conditions of unterminated high motivation are maintained over a period of time. This means that, according to the view proposed, the causal conditions that give rise to primary anxiety and those that evoke defensive processes are much the same. Primary anxiety is produced by unterminated high motivation; defensive processes are evoked when high motivation remains unterminated for a period of time.

A theory of this kind can predict correctly the temporal relations of anxiety and defence that are observed clinically. First, the experience of primary anxiety is expected to precede the onset of defensive processes. Secondly, as in due course these processes come largely to exclude and to immobilise the unterminated motivational system, a reduction of primary anxiety is to be expected. Thirdly, if subsequently defensive processes are reduced in degree, e.g. by analytic treatment, and the motivational system is thereby released from immobility, an outbreak of anxiety is once again to be expected.

The *temporal* relationship of anxiety to defence inherent in this theory is thus the conventional one. Where it differs is in its view of the *causal* relationship. Whilst anxiety precedes defensive process, it is not regarded as causing it. Instead, each is regarded as being the result of the same causal conditions, the one, anxiety, following at once, the other, defensive process, after an interval. Each is the result of unterminated high motivation.

Functions and consequences

The essential effect of defences that follow loss, it is argued, is to segregate one motivational system from another. The means whereby this is achieved, it is postulated, is the elaborate system of selective exclusion which is one of the major activities of the CNS. The next problem is to review the many consequences which result from this activity and to discriminate, so far as possible, those that, on balance, promote species survival from those that are either neutral or harmful to it. As already explained, to any that, on balance, promote it the term "function" is usually applied. That such occur provides an explanation of why in the course of evolution the process has been subject to positive selection and thus transmitted by heredity to the current generation. The remaining consequences can be understood as either the natural by-products of the process or, if harmful, the price that must be paid by the organism for being equipped with this particular process. Whilst, therefore, all functions are consequences, by no means all consequences are functions: on the contrary, some consequences are adverse to the organism and therefore pathological.

In order to establish this distinction, which is not always clear in psycho-analytic writing, let us consider two analogies – one physical, the other physiological.

In an airplane a particular instrument may, on balance, be of great value. This value explains why the plane is so equipped and is the function of the instrument. Carrying it, however, will have various other consequences, e.g. for instrument lay-out and operational procedures; most of these are likely to be incidental and neutral by-products. Certain other consequences, however, are adverse. Weight is always one such. Another is the possibility that, if the instrument fails in a certain way, its very failure may endanger the plane. Weight and the risk of a certain type of failure are the penalties inherent in carrying the instrument. In biological terms the risk of such failure may be described as the pathologic potential.

In a similar way we can analyse the consequences for an organism of its being equipped with a process which leads to a rise of temperature in conditions of infection. Certain of its consequences are beneficial; these consequences explain why in the course of evolution the organism has come to be so equipped; they are its functions. Other consequences, e.g. sweating and shivering, are only the by-products, neither beneficial nor adverse. If, however, the temperature rises above a certain point or continues for too long, adverse effects may outweigh the beneficial. The risk of such happening is the penalty inherent in the equipment and its pathological potential. This is a principle formulated a century ago by Claude Bernard and likely to be as relevant to psychopathology as to physiopathology.

In the light of this principle let us look afresh at the consequences of the defensive processes that follow loss. Earlier I suggested that a defensive process such as that described by Freud as primary repression, (and by Fairbairn and Melanie Klein as splitting) could hardly be considered advantageous. One of its effects, we know, is to leave the organism with two motivational systems "contrary to each other and independent of each other" (Freud, 1949). The ego "has certainly inhibited and damaged the particular part of the id concerned"; Freud remarks elsewhere:

but it has at the same time given it some independence and has renounced some of its own sovereignty... The repressed is now, as it were, an outlaw; it is excluded from the great organisation of the ego and is subject only to the laws which govern the realm of the unconscious.

(Freud, 1926d, p.152)

A vast array of symptoms affecting behaviour, mood and thought can, it is clear, be understood as due to the calamitous effects of the "unrealistic" and "irresponsible" activities of these outlaws.

Such effects, it seems likely, are unalloyedly adverse; consequences certainly, but not the functions of the processes concerned. That they may in certain conditions be their result is to be regarded as a risk and the pathologic potential of processes which, when acting in some more moderate way, are beneficial. If, therefore, we follow the principle of Bernard (1865, 1961), the task is to identify these potentially beneficial consequences, or in other words to identify the functions of the processes that, when operating adversely, result in primary repression.

In pursuing this search a major clue is to be found in Freud's reflections on the process of "isolation": "Even a normal person uses concentration to keep away not only what is irrelevant or unimportant, but, above all, what is unsuitable because it is contradictory" (Freud, 1926d, p.121). A great deal of the function of selective exclusion, it is contended, is to be understood in just these terms. The exclusion of what is irrelevant or unimportant, or at least believed to be so, is crucial to every effective integration and action. Without it an intolerable quantity of hotch potch information and incompatible motor repertoire would arrive in the integration pool, and efficient sorting prior to effective action would never be possible.

This is easy to understand. So, also, is the functional value of still further restricting information and motor repertoire in conditions of high motivation. When action is urgent it may be better to act less efficiently than to spend too long in deciding what to do – in exploring all avenues and leaving no stone unturned. Though the disadvantages of unconsidered and precipitate action are obvious, it is not difficult to see how, in the course of man's long evolution in primitive conditions, it has on balance been better to act fast than not to act at all.

Selection and exclusion, therefore, are essential for efficient action. On the basis of what criteria, we may next ask, do these processes do their selecting and how does the individual come by them? The main determinant for some, it seems clear, is genic action; for example, the neonate's preference for a female voice to other sounds and his preference a little later for complex visual patterns to simple ones (Fantz, 1961). For others, it seems equally plain, the main determinants are experience and learning. For this reason, and also because of the unfinished state of the young child's C.N.S., it is hardly surprising that in infancy and early childhood processes of selective exclusion work slowly and clumsily; or that, without appropriate experience (as in the case of individuals raised in a restricted environment), they may remain woefully inefficient.

Apart altogether from issues of this sort, however, there is one general property that seems inherent in these criteria that is of great relevance to my thesis. This property I shall term their "conservatism".

In a famous notebook entry Darwin remarked on the ease with which we forget data inconsistent with our theory. Every scientist knows how true this is and how the more intensely motivated he is to prove his point the less justice does he do his opponent's. If not carried too far, there is no great harm in this; harm comes mainly from pretending it is otherwise. But if in this respect even the trained scientist is a villain he is a saint compared to the ordinary man, and particularly to the ordinary child. By all odds the criteria which guide us in our acceptance and exclusion are extremely biased and extremely conservative. As Freud emphasised, what a normal person keeps away, above all, is what is *contradictory*.

If this is true, and I believe it self-evident, we are faced once more with the question what function does this property serve. In what way is such conservatism of selective criteria beneficial to the organism? How comes it to be of advantage that vast quantities of relevant information and of relevant motor patterns are subject to exclusion whilst much that is irrelevant accepted? Two reasons are readily discernible.

In the first place, it is evident that there is a limit to the sheer quantity of information and motor patterns that the integrative process can manage. Like the student who reads too undiscriminatingly and thereby develops a half-baked mind, an attempt to integrate too much can lead merely to chaos. For many purposes, better a little well-integrated than much more ill-digested. Striking the right balance is no easy task.

Quantity of information and of motor repertoire to be integrated is only one limiting factor, however. The other is its quality. For effective behaviour the individual needs coherent and self consistent schemas by which to organise both his input and his output. Contradictoriness, therefore, is itself a threat.

The danger to effective action that inheres simply in contradiction is perhaps too little recognised. To take account of information contradictory to the schemas with which we habitually operate is to become temporarily impotent. Every games player knows how disconcerting it is to attempt to relinquish a bad habit in order to acquire a better style. Temporarily his game will be even worse than it was before. Similarly, every lecturer knows how badly he presents material at a time when he is trying to recast his thoughts to take account of information that calls in question the theories he has hitherto so confidently taught. To utilise contradictory information requires the dissolution of existing schemas and the construction of new ones. Meanwhile performance suffers.

Whether or not it is of advantage to the individual to tolerate a period of disorganisation in order to organise afresh depends on circumstances. In a protected environment the balance of advantage may be favourable. But in an unprotected one it may not be so. On the contrary, to become disorganised, even temporarily, may make him impotent in a crisis and lead to disaster. In a state of nature conservatism may well be the lesser of two evils.

The hypothesis proposed, it will be seen, is a modification of Freud's idea that the function of primary repression is to preserve the organisation of the ego in conditions of excessive excitation or excessive instinctual demand. The process of primary repression, on this view, does not itself preserve the organisation of the ego in such conditions; indeed it tends to fracture it. Instead, it is seen as a special and pathological version of the process of selective exclusion that, in health, plays a key part in such organisation but which in conditions of unterminated high motivation may take a form that leads to adverse consequences. Although not identical with Freud's hypothesis, therefore, the one proposed is recognisably related to it.

With certain other of Freud's ideas the hypothesis conforms more closely. These ideas include the two principles of mental functioning, the pleasure and reality principles, and also the notion that a function of defensive process is to protect the ego from mental pain.

Behaviour determined by the pleasure principle, Tolman (1948) points out, can readily be equated with behaviour determined by a narrow cognitive map. When little information is accepted, the cognitive map is narrow and the resulting behaviour bull-headed: it is following the pleasure principle. When much information is accepted and integrated, on the other hand, the cognitive map is wide and the resulting behaviour better fitted to the circumstances: it is following the reality principle.

The hypothesis, moreover, accounts readily for the common observation that a motivational system that has been segregated tends to manifest itself in behaviour that follows the pleasure principle. Segregation, we know, tends to occur especially in early childhood when maps are narrow, and tends to occur, too, in conditions of high motivation when maps are narrower still. Any system so segregated, therefore, is not only bound to be narrowly organised at the start but, because thenceforward it lacks communication with other systems and is insulated from new information, is bound to remain so. In all these respects, therefore, the hypothesis advanced is consistent with empirical data and traditional theories.

It is consistent, too, with Freud's notion that defensive processes protect the ego from mental pain. The admission to the integrative process of contradictory information, it has been noted, may well lead performance to suffer. Not only that, but it may lead the performer himself to suffer also. Information of any sort that is incompatible with existing information, or motivation that is incompatible with existing motivation, is never welcome. To use and integrate it may require drastic reorganisation of existing schemas and systems; and inevitably this must be preceded by initial disorganisation. Such disorganisation, I have suggested (Bowlby, 1961), is always experienced as in some degree painful. The alternative and more frequent method of responding to incompatible information and motivation is to exclude it. By so doing disorganisation is made unnecessary and mental pain avoided.

On this hypothesis, therefore, the avoidance of mental pain is regarded as a consequence of the defensive process.[34] Whether or not on any one occasion exclusion of incompatible information and motivation is beneficial depends on the circumstances; the same is true of the concomitant avoidance of mental pain. Protection from mental pain, therefore, cannot be regarded as a function of defensive process. Instead, it is best regarded as a consequential by-product associated with processes which, depending on circumstances, vary from being beneficial to very pathogenic.

According to this hypothesis, it will be observed, a main criterion for determining whether information or motivation is to be excluded from integration is simply that it is incompatible with what is there already. If it proves adequate to explain the data, to search for other reasons why information or motivation is excluded becomes unnecessary; theories such as dread of the instincts or fear of the activity of the death instinct within become redundant. What grounds have we then for believing it to be adequate? For the limited task of explaining why defensive processes are habitually evoked by loss of a loved object, it is contended, there are grounds for thinking it probably is so.

Inevitably, loss of a loved object confronts the bereaved with information that is utterly incompatible with the schemas and systems hitherto active and dominant for him. To accept this information and to integrate it, therefore, requires the dissolution of these schemas and systems and their complete reorganisation. On the principle of conservatism, this is resisted. In place of the sequence acceptance, disorganisation, reorganisation there occur, instead, exclusion of incompatible information and maintenance of the status quo. Thus the existing set of schemas and systems based on the object's presence remains intact; whilst a second set based on its absence may begin to grow. If, therefore, the process of exclusion remains active, the individual grows up inhabited by two systems "contrary to each other and independent of each other".

---

34 [Bowlby notes:] In Learning Theory the fact that whenever a defensive process is reduced mental pain is experienced provides an explanation for its persisting: mental pain reinforces the process. In the theory proposed mental pain is not conceived as having this causal role.

Such, then, is the explanation offered for the tendency for defensive processes to follow loss. The tendency for them to persist is explicable on the same principles. Once a new system has become established, however inadequate and pathological it may be, it will tend to be self-perpetuating, accepting only what fits and excluding all else. This is the situation that confronts us when treating a sick patient. Information that fits existing schemas and systems, or can be distorted to fit, is accepted; what does not and cannot be made to fit is rejected. Thereby a potentially better reorganisation is sacrificed in favour of stability of whatever organisation happens to be dominant. Nowhere is the influence of vested interest more apparent.

Finally, let us compare this theory of defensive processes evoked by loss with those current in the literature.

Review of literature

It has been noted earlier that, especially from 1926 onwards, Freud adhered to the view that defences are of two sorts and arise in what are essentially two quite different situations. One sort is dependent on awareness of consequences, the other not; one sort results from learning, the other from trauma. In view of the task set in this paper, it is of special relevance that in all Freud's later writings the contexts in which the theory of primary repression is to be found show that he was still struggling to understand why patients tend to develop symptoms following trauma, which is the very problem that had first led him to the concept of defence. Thus the empirical basis for his later ideas is the same as that for his earlier ones.

It may now be noted that, amongst the traumatic factors with which Freud at both periods was concerned, is loss of object. In the *Studies on Hysteria* the reference is to "the irreparable loss of a loved person" (Freud, 1895d, p.10); in *Inhibitions, Symptoms and Anxiety* it is to the infant's "missing its mother"[35] (Freud, 1926d, p.170). In 1926, therefore, Freud reached a conclusion on the brink of which he had been thirty years earlier; amongst the commonest antecedents of the earliest and most fundamental repressions is loss of a loved figure.

Nevertheless, despite its being evident in all his later works that Freud identified the defences that follow loss with primary repression and processes related to it, few analysts have followed his lead. Instead, theories couched in teleological terms and invoking processes of secondary repression have been preferred. Almost always the ego is credited with awareness

---

35 [Bowlby notes:] Although loss of mother is regarded by Freud as usually constituting only a "danger situation", "if the infant happens at the time to be feeling a need which its mother should be the one of satisfy... it is a traumatic situation" (Freud, 1926d, p.170).

of the imminence of a painful or dangerous situation and with ability to take action to avoid it. Four analysts who have been deeply concerned with loss and the defences that follow it – Helene Deutsch, Melanie Klein, Edith Jacobson, and Fairbairn – all cast their formulations in this mould.

In her tentative attempt to account for the absence in some persons of grief following loss, Helene Deutsch (1937) postulates as "the motive power for the rejection of the emotion an inner awareness of inability to master emotion, that is, the awareness by the ego of its inadequacy". Edith Jacobson (1943) makes a different but equally teleological suggestion, namely that it is because of "disappointment and hostility" that the patient "tries to escape into a narcissistic withdrawal". A variant of this is adopted by Fairbairn (1943). The "quasi-independence" of the psychopath, he postulates, is "an attempt to convert his liabilities into assets.... He capitalised his insecurity and his inability to depend safely by renouncing all intimacy of social contact...." Although Melanie Klein's formulation (1940) is different again, it remains teleological. "The ego", she states, "is forced to develop methods of defence which are essentially directed against the 'pining' for the lost object". Whereas by other analysts such defences are seen as adverse to development, for Melanie Klein they are both inevitable and useful. These defences, she holds, "are fundamental to the whole ego-organisation" (Klein, 1948b, p.316). Nevertheless, the process may go too far. When early conflict and guilt are especially strong, she holds, there may be "a turning away from loved people or even... a rejection of them". There is a reason for this: "the fear that the loved person – to begin with the mother – may die because of the injuries inflicted upon her in phantasy.... makes it unbearable to be dependent upon this person" (Klein & Riviere, 1937).

In each of these formulations, it is seen, foresight in initiating defence and a purpose for achieving detachment are attributed to the ego; awareness of inability to master emotion, escape from repeated disappointment, fear of relying on a loved person who may die. In none of them is it easy, however, to distinguish what is thought to be cause and what function. Another difficulty is that none of these analysts presents evidence to support his particular hypothesis, nor are alternative explanations considered. More surprising, perhaps, is that none of them even refers to the concept of primary repression that Freud so clearly favoured in his later work when confronted with the problem of defences that follow loss.

In both its point of departure and its basic form the theory of defence advanced here resembles Freud's. Both start from notions of trauma and loss. In one passage Freud defines trauma as a situation in which "the ego comes into contact with excessive libidinal demand" (Freud, 1933a, p.123); for me it is a situation in which there is high motivation persisting over a period of time, a concept not very different. Not only do both theories make a clear distinction between causation and function but as regards the functions that it is thought defences serve there is substantial agreement.

There are, however, at least two key points at which my theorising about defence differs from Freud's. Reference has already been made to one of them – Freud's hypothesis that defence is a form of withdrawal modelled on the way we respond to painful stimuli assailing us from the outside world. The second concerns his concept of "excitation" as a quantity, with attributes resembling those of physical energy. It is a one which, ironically enough, sprang from his desire to give his theorising a sound scientific basis.

In their early work on hysteria, Breuer and Freud had emphasised three themes: trauma, repression of affect-laden memories, and abreaction. Theory had been cast in terms of the adequacy with which the affect aroused by trauma is discharged at the time of the trauma or remains in some way undischarged. This notion of affect Freud then linked with a purely physical model of the mental apparatus and its discharge, the "principle of constancy", with both of which he was then engrossed.[36] In this way he developed a form of theorising, in terms of the increase and decrease of a hypothetical energy, that has lived on to the present day. It is, however, a model that has many deficiencies. Not only has it been criticised by a number of analysts (e.g. Colby, 1955; Fairbairn, 1952), but it belongs to a larger class of theory, that of energy models of motivation, the shortcomings of which are now clearly defined.[37]

It is therefore of interest to note that, had Freud been less eager to adopt a model of the mental apparatus based on physical concepts, data for a model based on biological and psychological concepts were already in his possession. It is experiences that are not adequately responded to at the time they occur, he had observed, that seem to give rise to later psychological trouble. Provided there is an "adequate reaction", ill-effects seem to be avoided. The "adequate reactions" to which he pointed as examples, which include "crying oneself out" and "acts of revenge" (Freud, 1895d, p.8), turn out, however, to be differentiated and highly structured sequences of behaviour, each with its own peculiar motivation. To describe them all simply as "discharges of affect" conceals these facts. In a form that more closely fits his data, the conclusions which Freud had reached may be reformulated as follows: (a) there are situations in which specifically motivated behaviour and its accompanying affect is in some degree evoked but remains not only unexpressed but unknown to the subject; (b) the conditions in which this occurs are characterised by very high motivation in circumstances

36 [Bowlby notes:] See Strachey's Editor's *Introduction to Studies in Hysteria* (Freud, 1895d, pp.18–25).
37 [Bowlby notes:] See the carefully reasoned paper by Hinde (1960).

where it cannot be acted upon, and the accompanying affect is at a correspondingly high degree of intensity.

The truth is that quantities of excitation, their damming up and their discharge, are theoretical constructs far removed from the observations which Freud had made and which analysts in the therapeutic situation continue to make. Constructs such as motivation to perform specific sequences or classes of behaviour and directed towards specific objects are much nearer to them. This is true also of the observations on separated children that are my concern in this series of papers. In the theory of defence I have proposed, motivation and behaviour rather than affect and its discharge are the basic concepts.

References

Ainsworth, M. D. S., & Ainsworth, L. H. (1958). *Measuring Security in Personal Adjustment*. Toronto: University of Toronto Press.

Bahrick, H. P., Fitts, P. M., & Rankin, R. E. (1952). Effect of incentives upon reactions to peripheral stimuli. *Journal of Experimental Psychology*, *44*: 400–440.

Bahrick, H. P., Noble, M., & Fitts, P. M. (1954). Extra-task performance as a measure of learning a primary task. *Journal of Experimental Psychology*, *48*: 298–302.

Barber, T. X. (1958). The concept of hypnosis. *Journal of Psychology*, *45*: 115–131.

Bartlett, F.C. (1932). *Remembering: A Study in Experimental and Social Psychology*. Cambridge: Cambridge University Press.

Bernard, C. (1865, 1961). *An Introduction to the Study of Experimental Medicine*. Transl. H. C. Greene. New York: Collier.

Birch, H. G. (1945). The role of motivational factors in insightful problem-solving. *Journal of Comparative Psychology*, *38*: 295–317.

Bowlby, J. (1960). Separation anxiety. *International Journal of Psycho-Analysis*, *41*: 89–113.

Bowlby, J. (1961). Processes of mourning. *International Journal of Psycho-Analysis*, *42*: 317–334.

Bowlby, J. (1963). Pathological mourning and childhood mourning. *Journal of the American Psychoanalytic Association*, *11*: 500–541.

Brenner, C. (1957). The nature and development of the concept of repression in Freud's writings. *The Psychoanalytic Study of the Child*, *12*: 19–46.

Breuer, J., & Freud, S. (1895d). *Studies on Hysteria. S. E. 2*. London: Hogarth Press.

Bruner, J. S., Matter, J., & Papanek, M. L. (1955). Breadth of learning as a function of drive level and mechanization. *Psychological Review*, *62*: 1–10.

Burlingham D. & Freud, A. (1942). *Young Children in War-time*. Oxford: Allen & Unwin.

Cobb, S. (1952). On the nature and locus of mind. *Archives of Neurology and Psychiatry*, *67*: 172–177.

Colby, K. M. (1955). *Energy and Structure in Psychoanalysis*. New York: Ronald Press.

Deutsch, H. (1937). Absence of grief. *Psychoanalytic Quarterly*, *6*: 12–22.

Deutsch, J. A. (1953). A new type of behaviour theory. *British Journal of Psychology*, *44*: 304–317.

Deutsch, J. A. (1960). *Structural Basis of Behaviour*. London: Cambridge University Press.

Dollard, J., & Miller, N. E. (1950). *Personality and Psychotherapy: An Analysis in Terms of Learning, Thinking, and Culture.* New York: McGraw Hill.

Eriksen, C. W., & Browne, C. T. (1956). An experimental and theoretical analysis of perceptual defense. *The Journal of Abnormal and Social Psychology, 52*: 224–230.

Erikson, E. (1954). The dream specimen of psychoanalysis. *Journal of the American Psychoanalytic Association, 2*: 5–56.

Fairbairn, W.R.D. (1943). The return of the bad object (with special reference to the "War Neurosis"). In: W.R.D. Fairbairn, *Psychoanalytical Studies of the Personality* (pp. 55–81). London: Routledge.

Fairbairn, W.R.D. (1952). *Psychoanalytical Studies of the Personality.* London: Tavistock Press.

Fantz, R. L. (1961). The origin of form perception. *Scientific American, 204*: 66–73.

Fenichel, O. (1945). *The Psychoanalytic Theory of Neurosis.* New York: Norton.

Fessard, A. (1954). Mechanisms of nervous integration and conscious experience. In: E. D. Adrian, F. Bremer, & H. H. Jasper (eds.), *Brain Mechanisms and Consciousness* (pp. 200–237). Oxford: Blackwell.

French, T. M. (1938). Defense and synthesis in the function of the ego—Some observations stimulated by Anna Freud's "The Ego and the Mechanisms of Defense". *Psychoanalytic Quarterly, 7*: 537–553.

Freud, A. (1936). *Ego and the Mechanisms of Defence.* London: Hogarth Press.

Freud, S. (1893a). *On the Psychical Mechanism of Hysterical Phenomena.* [with J. Breuer] *S. E., 2*: 3–17. London: Hogarth Press.

Freud, S. (1894a). *The Neuro-Psychoses of Defence. S. E., 3*: 157–185. London: Hogarth Press.

Freud, S. (1895d). *Studies on Hysteria.* [with J. Breuer]. *S. E. 2.* London: Hogarth Press.

Freud, S. (1900a). *The Interpretation of Dreams. S. E., 4–5*: 633–685. London: Hogarth Press.

Freud, S. (1901b). *The Psychopathology of Everyday Life. S. E., 6.* London: Hogarth Press.

Freud, S. (1905c). *Jokes and their Relation to the Unconscious. S. E., 8.* London: Hogarth Press.

Freud, S. (1914d). *On the History of the Psycho-Analytic Movement. S. E., 14*: 3–66. London: Hogarth Press.

Freud, S. (1915d). *Repression. S. E., 14*: 143–158. London: Hogarth Press.

Freud, S. (1916–1917). *Introductory Lectures on Psycho-Analysis. 1916–1917. S. E., 15–16.* London: Hogarth Press.

Freud, S. (1920g). *Beyond the Pleasure Principle. S. E., 18*: 7–64. London: Hogarth Press.

Freud, S. (1925d). *An Autobiographical Study. S. E., 20*: 3–70. London: Hogarth Press.

Freud, S. (1926d). *Inhibitions, Symptoms and Anxiety. S. E., 20*: 77–174. London: Hogarth Press.

Freud, S. (1926f [1925]). *Psycho-Analysis. S. E., 20*: 260–269. London: Hogarth Press.

Freud, S. (1933a). *New Introductory Lectures on Psycho-Analysis. S. E., 22*: 3–182. London: Hogarth Press.

Freud, S. (1939a). *Moses and Monotheism. S. E., 23*: 3–137. London: Hogarth Press.

Freud, S. (1940). An outline of psycho-analysis. *International Journal of Psycho-Analysis, 21*: 27–84.

Freud, S. (1940a [1938]). *An Outline of Psycho-Analysis. S. E., 23*: 141–207. London: Hogarth Press.

Freud, S. (1949). *An Outline of Psychoanalysis.* Oxford: W. W. Norton.

Hampshire, S. (1962). Disposition and memory. *International Journal of Psycho-Analysis, 43*: 59–68.

Harlow, H. F. (1952). Learning. *Annual Review of Psychology, 3*: 29–54.

Harlow, H. F. (1953). Mice, monkeys, men, and motives. *Psychological Review, 60*: 23–35.

Hartmann, H. (1939). *Ego Psychology and the Problem of Adaptation.* New York: International Universities Press.

Hernandez-Peon, R., & Hagbarth, K. (1955a). Interaction between afferent and cortically induced reticular responses. *Journal of Neurophysiology, 8*: 44–55.

Hernandez-Peon, R., & Scherrer, H. (1955b). Habituation to acoustic stimuli in cochlear nucleus. *Federation Proceedings of American Societies for Experimental Biology, 14*: 71.

Hinde, R. A. (1959). Motivation. *IBIS, International Journal of Avian Science, 101*: 353–357.

Hinde, R. A. (1960). Energy models of motivation. *Symposium of the Society of Experimental Biology, 14*: 199–213.

Hull, C. L. (1943). *Principles of Behavior.* New York: Appleton-Century.

Jacobson, E. (1943). Depression, the Oedipus Complex in the development of depressive mechanisms. *Psychiatric Quarterly, 12*: 541–560.

Jahoda, M. (1958). *Current Concepts of Positive Mental Health.* Joint Commission on Mental Illness and Health, Monograph Series No. 1. New York: Basic Books.

Janis, I. L. (1958). *Psychological Stress: Psychoanalytic and Behavioral Studies of Surgical Patients.* New York: Wiley.

Klein, M. (1932). *The Psychoanalysis of Children.* London: Hogarth Press.

Klein, M. (1940). Mourning and its relationship to manic-depressive states. *International Journal of Psychoanalysis, 21*: 125–153.

Klein, M. (1948a). A contribution to the theory of anxiety and guilt. *International Journal of Psychoanalysis, 29*: 113–123.

Klein, M. (1948b). *Contributions to Psychoanalysis, 1921–1945.* London: Hogarth Press.

Klein, M. (1952). The origins of transference. *International Journal of Psychoanalysis, 33*: 433–438.

Klein, M. (1957). *Envy and Gratitude: A Study of Unconscious Forces.* New York: Basic Books.

Klein, M., Heimann, P., Isaacs, S., & Riviere, J. (1952). *Developments in Psycho-Analysis.* London: Hogarth Press.

Klein, M., & Riviere, J. (1937). *Love, Hate and Reparation.* London: Hogarth Press.

Kuffler, S. W. (1953). Discharge patterns and functional organization of mammalian retina. *Journal of Neurophysiology, 16*: 37–68.

Lambercier, M., & Rey, A. (1935). Contribution à l'étude de l'intelligence pratique chez l'enfant [Contribution to the study of practical intelligence in children]. *Archives de Psychologie, 25*: 1–59.

Lewin, B. D. (1950). *The Psychoanalysis of Elation.* New York: Norton.

Liddell, H. S. (1956). *Emotional Hazards in Animals and Man*. Springfield, IL: Thomas.

Livingston, R. B. (1959). Central control of receptors and sensory transmission systems. In J. Field (ed.) *Handbook of Physiology, Section. I. Neurophysiology* (pp. 741–760). Washington, D.C.: American Physiological Society.

Livingston, R. B., & Hernandez-Peon, R. (1955). Somatic functions of the nervous system. *Annual Review of Physiology, 17*: 269–292.

Luria, A. R. (1932). *The Nature of Human Conflicts or Emotion, Conflict and Will. An Objective Study of Disorganisation and Control of Human Behaviour*. New York: Grove Press.

Magoun, H. (1958). *The Waking Brain*. Springfield, IL: Thomas.

Masserman, J. H. (1943). *Behaviour and Neurosis*. Chicago: Chicago University Press.

Melzack, R., Stotler, W. A., & Livingston, W. K. (1958). Effects of discrete brain lesions in cats on perception of noxious stimulation. *Journal of Neurophysiology, 21*: 353–367.

Miller, D. R., & Swanson, G. E. (1960). *Inner Conflicts and Defence*. New York: Holt.

Nissen, H. W. (1954). The nature of the drive as innate determinant of behaviour organisation. *Nebraska Symposium on Motivation*, pp 308–309.

Olds, J. (1958). Satiation effects in self-stimulation of the brain. *Journal of Comparative and Physiological Psychology, 51*: 675–678.

Paramonova, N. P. (1956). On the formation of interactions between the two signal systems in the normal child. In: A. R. Luria (ed.), *Problems of the Higher Nervous Activity of the Normal and Abnormal Child, Vol 1* (pp. 18–83). Moscow: Pedagological Science Press.

Peters, R. S. (1958). *The Concept of Motivation*. London: Routledge & Kegan Paul.

Pittendrigh, C. S. (1958). Perspectives in the study of biological clocks. In *Symposium on Perspectives in Marine Biology*, pp. 239–268. Berkeley: University of California Press.

Postman, L., Bruner, J. S., & McGinnies, E. (1948). Personal values as selective factors in perception. *The Journal of Abnormal and Social Psychology, 43*: 142–154.

Pribram, K. H. (1960). A review of theory in physiological psychology. *Annual Review of Psychology, 11*: 1–40.

Rapaport, D. (1953). On the psycho-analytic theory of affects. *International Journal of Psycho-Analysis, 34*: 177–198.

Schaffer, H. R. (1954). Behaviour under stress: a neurophysiological hypothesis. *Psychological Review, 61*: 323–333.

Schneirla, T. C. (1959). An evolutionary and developmental theory of biphasic processes underlying approach and withdrawal. In: M. R. Jones (ed.), *Nebraska Symposium on Motivation* (pp. 1–42). Oxford: University of Nebraska Press.

Scott, J. (1949). The relative importance of social and hereditary factors in producing disturbances in life adjustment during periods of stress in laboratory animals. *Research publications-Association for Research in Nervous and Mental Disease, 29*: 61–71.

Scott, J. P. (1957). Animal and human children. *Children, 4*: 163–168.

Scott, J. P. (1958). *Animal Behaviour*. Chicago: University of Chicago Press.

Sperling, S. J. (1958). On denial and the essential nature of defence. *International Journal of Psych-Analysis, 39*: 25–38.

Sperry, R. W. (1945). The problem of the central nervous system reorganisation after nerve regeneration and muscle transposition: A critical review. *Quarterly Review of Biology, 20*: 311–369.

Sperry, R. W. (1950). Neuronal specificity. In: P. Weiss (ed.), *Genetic Neurology* (pp. 232–239). Chicago: University of Chicago Press.

Thompson, W. R., & Heron, W. (1954). The effects of restricting early experience on the problem-solving capacity of dogs. *Canadian Journal of Psychology, 8*: 17–31.

Tolman, E. C. (1948). Cognitive maps in rats and men. *Psychological Review, 55*: 189–208.

Vince, M. A. (1958). String-pulling in birds. II. Differences related to age in green-finches, chaffinches, and canaries. *Animal Behaviour, 6*: 53–59.

Vince, M. A. (1961). Developmental changes in learning capacity. In: W. H. Zangwill (ed.), *Current Problems in Animal Behaviour* (pp. 225–247). Cambridge: Cambridge University Press.

Weiss, P. (1950). Some aspects of neural growth, regeneration, and function. In: P. Weiss (ed.), *Genetic Neurology: Problems of Development, Growth and Regeneration of the Nervous System and its Functions* (pp. 199–207). Chicago: University of Chicago Press.

Weiss, P. (1955). Nervous system, (neurogenesis). In: B. H. Willier, P. Weiss, & V. Hamburger (eds.), *Analysis of Development* (pp. 346–401). Philadelphia: Saunders.

Weiss, P. A., & Brown, P. F. (1941). Electromyographic studies on recoordination of leg movements in poliomyelitis patients with transposed tendons. *Proceedings, Society for Experimental Biological Medicine, 48*: 284–287.

Zeigarnik, B. V. (1927). Das Behalten erledigter und unerledigter Handlungen (Remembering completed and uncompleted tasks). *Psychologische Forschung (Psychological Research), 9*: 1–85.

Appendix

SELECTIVE EXCLUSION & LEVELS OF MOTIVATION[38]

Motivation	Exclusion
Level 1. LOW	Slight e.g. day dreaming free-association
Level 2. MODERATE	Moderate Some degree of concentration but still possible to attend to other input
Level 3. HIGH	Considerable Strong concentration & resulting exclusion of all other input
Level 4. VERY HIGH (? or persistence of high)	Erratic Whilst exclusion continues on a considerable scale, there is also a tendency for responses to a wider class of objects than in other conditions of motivation (cf Hinde) cf Vacuum Response - Parkes

38 [Editors' note:] This is a diagram compiled from a contemporaneous note: Bowlby, J. Theory of Defence, JB notes, 1960-63. PP/BOW/H10

SELECTIVE EXCLUSION & LEVELS OF MOTIVATION.

Motivation   Exclusion

Level 1. ~~High~~ LOW   Slight
eg. day- dreaming
free - association

Level 2   MODERATE   Moderate
Some degree of concentration
but still possible to attend
to other input

Level 3   HIGH   Considerable
Strong concentration &
resulting exclusion of
all other input

Level 4   VERY HIGH   Erratic
(? or persisting high)   Whilst exclusion continues
on a considerable scale, there
is also a tendency for
responses to be made to a
wider class of objects than
in other conditions of motivation
(cf Hride).

cf Vacuum Response - Parkes

Theory of Defence, JB notes, 1960-63. PP/BOW/H10

Chapter 2

Loss, detachment and defence

October 1962 [Editors: Wellcome Collection Archive PP/BOW/D.3/69-70]
[Bowlby] Note: This paper will likely be the final chapter of a book provisionally entitled *The Psychopathology of Loss*.

Introduction

In the preceding paper of this series *Pathological Mourning and Childhood Mourning* (Bowlby, 1962) I described four pathological patterns of mourning that are to be found in adults and compared them with the patterns of response that are known to be typical of infants and young children following loss. The conclusion drawn was that the two sets of patterns are substantially the same; in other words, that the mourning responses that are commonly seen in infancy bear many of the features that are the hallmarks of pathological mourning in the adult. Both, it was found, are characterised by the onset of defensive processes which have the effect either of rendering yearning for the lost object and also reproach against it unconscious, or else of splitting the ego into two parts – one organised on the basis of the object's being irretrievably lost, the other on the basis of its being recoverable. Although inevitably the discussion raised a number of basic problems regarding defence, because it was mainly at a descriptive level there was no opportunity to examine them properly. In this paper and the next ones, therefore, I shall attempt to make good this omission.

In keeping with the task in hand the point of departure will again be the behaviour to be observed in young children during a period of separation from mother. Since it is the third phase of this behaviour, that of detachment, that poses the problem of defence, the first issue to be considered will be how this kind of behavior is best to be understood. There are three main hypotheses current: that it is due to a withdrawal of libido and therefore not to a defensive process: that it is due to defensive processes originating during the period of separation itself; that, although due to defensive processes, these do not originate during separation but are to be traced to faulty development that has already occurred in an earlier phase, especially during the first year of life. The conclusion that will be drawn is that such evidence as we have favours the second hypothesis, namely that detached behaviour is due to the effects of defensive processes that originate during the period of separation itself.

Although at variance with the formulations of some prominent analysts, this conclusion is consonant with many of Freud's ideas on the problem of defence. Just as in an earlier paper (Bowlby, 1961) it was emphasised that anxiety following separation was often at the heart of Freud's thinking on the problem of anxiety, so will it be seen, when the literature is examined, that defence following loss was often at the centre of his thinking about defence. A reading of *Studies on Hysteria* (Freud, 1895d), of *Inhibitions, Symptoms and Anxiety* (Freud, 1926d) and some of his later papers (e.g., Freud, 1927 [1940]) shows that repression, splitting of the ego and denial are each traced by him to the experience of loss. Other analysts, too, have recognised that a common condition in which these defences are evoked is loss of a loved object. Thus, although hardly a commonplace, there is nothing novel in the conclusion that defensive processes may have their origin during a period of separation occurring in the early years.

Even so it is a conclusion that by implication calls in question hypotheses regarding the determinants of pathological mourning that have been long and strongly held. This other hypothesis, it will be shown, is consistent with what is known of the personality structure of individuals prone to respond to loss with pathological mourning and also with the conclusions that were reached in an earlier paper (Bowlby, 1960a) regarding the origin of separation anxiety of pathological degree.

Detachment: three hypotheses

Of the theoretical problems raised by the behaviour shown by young children when they are separated from their mothers, those of defence are posed by the behaviour Robertson and I have termed Detachment. This, it will be remembered, is characteristic of the third of the three phases of response to separation that have been delineated, of which the first two are those of Protest and Despair. Since the whole of my argument turns on the outcome of empirical observations, it may be useful to describe them briefly again.

Whereas in the phase of protest the child is in a state of acute distress and seeking frantically to recover his mother, and in the phase of Despair one of hopelessness about his success in doing so, in the phase of Detachment he seems no longer to be preoccupied with his missing mother and instead to be "settling down" to the new conditions. This is often welcomed by those caring for him as a sign that he is himself again. In words derived from Robertson's reports: "He no longer rejects the nurses, accepts their care and the food and toys they bring and may even smile and be sociable". This is only a half of the picture, however:

> When his mother visits ... it can be seen that all is not well, for there
> is a striking absence of the behaviour characteristic of the strong
> attachment normal at this age. So far from greeting his mother he may
> seem hardly to know her; so far from clinging to her he may remain
> remote and apathetic; instead of tears there is a listless turning away.
> He seems to have lost all interest in her.
>
> (Bowlby, 1960a, p.28)

This description is based on the observations made by Robertson in
1948–1951, and later confirmed by Heinicke.[1] These observations were preceded, however, by those made in the Hampstead Nurseries during the war
by Dorothy Burlingham and Anna Freud (Burlingham & A. Freud, 1942).
Since their findings are identical with the later ones, it is of interest to
quote them; so far as I know, apart from the single case reported by
Helene Deutsch (1919), this was the first occasion that attention was
drawn to the behaviour following loss in early childhood that we describe
as Detachment. Of children under three years of age they write:

> That the shock of parting at this stage is really serious is further
> proved by the observation that a number of these children fail to rec-
> ognise their mothers when they visit after they have 'settled down' in
> the new surroundings. The mothers themselves realise that this lack of
> recognition is not due to any limitation of the faculty of memory as
> such. The same child who looks at his mother's face with stony indif-
> ference as if she were a complete stranger, will have no difficulty in rec-
> ognising lifeless objects which have belonged to his past. When taken
> home again he will recognise the rooms, the position of the beds, and
> will remember the contents of the cupboards etc.
>
> (Burlingham & A. Freud, 1942)

Usually such children respond more readily to their fathers and other figures. A striking example of such a differential response was described to
me by a mother: a little girl of three, on returning home from hospital
after a two months stay unvisited, remained aloof from all members of the
family except the dog, which she welcomed.

Though the validity of these data is now well-established, their interpretation remains a matter of acute controversy. As already noted, there are
current at present three hypotheses to account for the processes that underlie detached behaviour. Set out more fully they are –

---

1 [Bowlby notes:] See Robertson and Bowlby (1952), Robertson (Robertson, 1953b April),
  Bowlby & Robertson (in preparation), [Editors' note: possibly their paper of 1956], Heinicke
  (1956), Heinicke and Westheimer (1961).

1. Detached behaviour is due not to the effects of defensive processes but to a withdrawal of libido. This view has recently been advanced by Anna Freud (1960).
2. Detached behaviour is due to the effects of defensive processes which originate during the period of separation (loss) itself. This is a view advanced by Freud (Freud, 1893a, 1926d, 1927 [1940], 1938 [1940])) and by Helene Deutsch (1937), Lindemann (1944) and Bowlby (1954).
3. Although detached behaviour is due to the effects of defensive processes, these processes have not originated during the current period of separation (loss) but are to be attributed to processes originating earlier, in particular as a result of faulty development in the early months of life. This view is implicit in the work of Abraham (1924) and Rado (1928), and has been made explicit in that of Melanie Klein (1940).

Let us start with the first hypothesis.

In her comments on an earlier paper of mine, Anna Freud (1960) dissents from the view that defensive processes underlie the condition of detachment. In its place she advances the hypothesis that the condition is due to withdrawal of libido from the object. In arguing her case, she starts by calling in question my use of a term[2] that implies:

> a defensive process directed either against the recognition of external reality (i.e., the absence of the mother), or against the affect itself (i.e., an intolerably painful sense of bereavement). In neither case", she continues, "does it include the purely libidinal aspect which seems of the greatest importance to us. If we see the trauma of separation from the mother in terms of what happens to the libidinal cathexis of her image, we take the phases of protest and despair as manifestations of the child's attempt to maintain the libidinal tie with the absent object, the third phase as a sign that cathexis is not denied but actually withdrawn from the object.
>
> (A. Freud, 1960, p.3)

Selecting her terms to fit this theoretical model she proposes:

> the use of the term '*withdrawal*' for [the] third phase of bereavement behaviour. It has the advantage of covering the manifest withdrawn

---

2 [Bowlby notes:] Although in her comments Anna Freud is referring to my earlier formulation in which I employed the term "denial" instead of "detachment", the change of term does not materially alter the burden of her criticism.

behaviour of the child as well as the internal process of libido withdrawal by which we believe this behaviour to be caused.

(A. Freud, 1960, p.3)

Plainly there is a divergence between us. Whereas in this formulation Anna
Freud holds that there is a withdrawal of cathexis from the mother's image,
to me the evidence points to a persistence of the cathexis, combined with
a strong defensive process (in the terminology she uses "counter-cathexis")
which leads to its becoming unconscious. This evidence is of three main
kinds.

First, there is the way that, after a separation lasting a few weeks, the
child responds to his mother following reunion with her. Were Anna
Freud's recent formulation to be correct, it would be expected that his
attachment to his mother would develop again only gradually. This however, is not the case. As a rule, after a period during which such detachment as has developed persists, his old attachment manifests itself with
extreme intensity. He refuses to let go of his mother and throws a tantrum
every time he loses sight of her. Plainly his urge to attach himself to her
has not faded during the separation; rather has it remained latent within
him. After reunion it is active again and with increased force. This is all
the more impressive when, as in some children, the change from detachment to attachment is sudden.

A second type of evidence that points strongly to defensive processes
being at work is the way that, after it is over, some young children refer, or
fail to refer, to the separation experience. Even after only short stays away
from home, some of them either do not speak of the experience or deny its
painfulness. For example, on the day of her return from hospital, Laura,
who had been acutely unhappy and had been sobbing unbrokenly for
a couple of hours before her mother's arrival to take her home, claimed
blandly that she had had a "nice holiday". Another example of the same
reaction is the explanation of his loss proffered by the two-year-old Rudi,
the subject of Helene Deutsch's (1919) report. Utterly miserable three days
after the departure of a nurse who had been his mother- figure, Rudi nonetheless explained her absence by alleging "with an air of greatest indifference 'she went to the tailor'".

The third type of evidence that points to the activity of defensive processes is the way that, later on, some young children respond to persons
and places associated with their experience. For example, a month after her
return from hospital Laura with her mother met Mr. Robertson in the
street. Although during her eight days away she had got to know him
extremely well, now she denied all knowledge of him.

That observations of this sort are not trivial is shown by a number of
others. Observations made by Robertson during a return visit to hospital
of a boy of four and a half years are dramatic but not atypical. Roddy had

been thirteen months old when admitted to hospital on account of tuber-culosis and had remained there three years. Naturally during that time, he had got to know the ward sister and many of the children very well indeed. Nevertheless, when he returned there six months after discharge, he claimed that he had never seen the hospital nor met any of the staff and children before. Nor did his behaviour suggest he was shamming. The chil-dren with whom he had lived for so long recognised him and called him by name, and the ward sister greeted him warmly; but he acted towards them as if they had been strangers. Apart from an unwanted silence, the only glimmer of recognition he betrayed in the course of a visit lasting over an hour was for the dining hall. On return home again, except to say he had been for a ride in a car, he made no reference to the visit. It was as though he had two lives and an iron curtain separated one from the other.

Not all young children show this failure to recognise and respond to fig-ures and places associated with the separation nor are all of them either silent about the experience or inclined to brush it off lightly. Thus only a proportion of children (though probably a substantial proportion) show behaviour constituting the second and third types of evidence of defence. Evidence of the first type, on the other hand, is prolific. In almost every case of short separation of which we know there is, after reunion, intense and anxious clinging to mother. The only exceptions are children who before separation were not attached and those whose separations have been so prolonged and/or repeated that the state of detachment persists.

On the basis of evidence of these three types it is concluded that, during separation, defensive processes are undoubtedly at work. It is therefore of interest to find that in an earlier publication (jointly with Dorothy Burling-ham, Burlingham & A. Freud, 1942), Anna Freud has herself taken this view. After having given the description (already quoted) of the detached behaviour of children under three years of age who were left in the nursery by their mothers, Dorothy Burlingham and Anna Freud offer an explan-ation of it:

> Failure to recognise the mother occurs when something has happened to the image of the mother in the child's mind, i.e., to its inner rela-tionship to her. The mother has disappointed the child and left his longing for her unsatisfied: so he turns against her with resentment and *rejects the memory of her person from his consciousness.*
>
> (p.57, my italics)

A little later, when contrasting the behaviour of slightly older children with that of these younger ones, they term the process "complete repression". "After three years of age children will not normally forget their parents. Their memories are more stable, change of attitude takes the place of *com-plete repression*" (p.57, my italics).

Moreover, they record the view that even in these older children a partial repression occurs. Whereas positive feelings may remain conscious, they remark, the negative feelings "undergo repression and create all sorts of moods and problems of behaviour" (Burlingham & A. Freud, 1942, p.64).

At this point a note on terminology may be useful. Although there is no reason to doubt that the term "repression", used by Dorothy Burlingham and Anna Freud, is the correct one to describe some, at least, of the defensive processes at work in the separated child, it is common for analysts to challenge it. For example, in a discussion following a showing of the film of Laura (Robertson, 1953a) and an exposition of some of Robertson's observations, several analysts maintained that what was described could not be due to repression. They suggested instead that it was due to denial or scotomization. I was not convinced and, after looking up the literature, wrote a note for the published version of the conference proceedings (Bowlby, 1954). Since I see no reason to modify my conclusions and since the arguments I then used still stand, I repeat them:

"We believe we are using the term 'repression' according to the traditional psychoanalytic usage, to indicate the removal from consciousness of ideas, affects and impulses which are felt to be painful or dangerous. Freud in his paper on *Repression* (Freud, 1915d) states that the essence of repression lies simply in the function of keeping something out of consciousness. This remains its standard usage (Hinsie & Shatsky, 1940)

"We do not believe that either 'denial' or 'scotomization' are correct terms to describe the basic processes observed. The term 'denial' seems first to have been used by Freud in his paper on *Negation* (Freud, 1925h). He notes that something which is repressed may appear in consciousness in the form of a negative (e.g., 'Well, it was certainly not my mother'), and argues that to deny is basically the same as to admit that it is something one would rather repress. A negative judgment is thus the intellectual substitute for repression. In his paper on *Fetishism* (Freud, 1927) Freud is very outspoken about Laforgue's introduction of the term 'to scotomize', remarking that a new term is justified only when it describes a new fact or brings it into prominence. But 'repression', he emphasises, is not only the oldest word in our psychoanalytical technology but one that already refers to this pathological process. If we wish to differentiate between the *idea* and the *affect*, he continues, it is permissible to limit the use of the term 'repression' to the affect and to use the term 'denial' when we mean the idea.

"Since", I concluded, "our observations show that the child's affect is greatly involved in the defensive process set in train by separation, together with his impulses to relate to his mother, it is clear that the term 'repression' is the right one to denote it. However, when a child purposefully avoids his mother and says he does not wish to be with her, the term 'denial' is evidently appropriate."

(Bowlby, 1954, p. 73)[3]

In this note I did not refer to "splitting of the ego" as a defensive process that follows loss because we have no evidence regarding it derived from direct observations of separated children. Nevertheless, as I make clear in an earlier paper (Bowlby, 1962), there is plenty of evidence that it occurs. Thus we find that repression, denial and splitting can all follow loss, which raises the question of how they are related to one another. Since this is one of the basic problems in the theory of defence its consideration will be postponed to a later paper. Meanwhile it is time to return to the theme of this section, the comparative merits of the three hypotheses regarding the nature of detachment.

On the basis of the evidence described, it is concluded, the first hypothesis regarding the nature of detachment must be ruled out; during separation, defensive processes, in particular repression, denial and splitting, are undoubtedly at work. The next question that arises is: do these processes originate during the period of separation itself, the second hypothesis, or are they to be attributed to faulty development that has preceded the experience, the third hypothesis? There are many analysts, for example Helene Deutsch, Edith Jacobson, Margaret Mahler and, by implication, Freud himself, who favour the second hypothesis; loss represents a trauma and evokes defence. Melanie Klein and her associates, however, have identified themselves with the third; in their opinion defensive processes of the kind described occur only in children whose development is already impaired. Although many analysts avoid committing themselves, the frequent emphasis on the importance of primary narcissism and the oral phase leads a number to a position which in this respect is not unlike that of Melanie Klein.

Since the issue is an empirical one, it can be settled only by evidence. The question to be decided is whether the occurrence of defensive processes leading to detachment is confined to children whose development is already impaired, as Melanie Klein and other analysts claim, or whether they are to be observed in all or at least a wide array of children of different, including satisfactory, development. Such evidence as we have does not favour the Kleinian and related hypotheses. In the first place the only young children of whom we have records who respond to a period of

---

3 [Bowlby notes:] Although I have made minor revisions in phraseology, this passage is little changed from the Note published in 1954 (p.73) and is therefore placed in quotation marks.

separation in an atypical way are those who, through previous separations or gross rejection, already have a most unsatisfactory relation to their mother: such children may appear almost unaffected by the change of environment. All the others respond with greater or less degrees of protest and despair, and later show typical detachment. It is possible, of course, that every child of whom we have records had had an impaired earlier development. Admittedly, since our data are inadequate, we cannot prove the contrary. On the other hand, certain of these children, for example some who have been removed to hospital although never particularly ill, appear to have had excellent relations with their mothers beforehand and to have been developing favourably. Thus, such evidence as we have supports the view that defensive processes arise *ab initio* during the course of separation, and does not favour a view that demands that the child's personality should already have been impaired by faulty development at an earlier phase.

When in the course of scientific discussion Robertson and I have presented our observations and the inferences we draw from them, their validity has constantly been challenged. It has been represented, for instance, that we have given too little weight to the fact that the children observed have not only lost their mothers but that some of them have been in the frightening surroundings of hospital, that some have been unwell, that some have had mothers who were pregnant and others of them mothers whose attitude was unfavourable. In meeting these representations, we have pointed out that children who are in residential nurseries, who are healthy and whose mothers are not pregnant behave in substantially the same way, so that these three conditions, whilst not of negligible importance, cannot be regarded as the main determinants of the behaviour with which we are concerned. To assess the significance of the fourth variable, the child's previous development is, as already stated, far more difficult, and we make no claim to have done so with any certainty. On the other hand, we know of no positive evidence to support the view that it is only when previous development has gone astray that the child responds to separation with detachment.

In evaluating criticism of the kind described it should be borne in mind, first, that, apart from Dorothy Burlingham and Anna Freud, few analysts have published direct observations of their own on how young children respond to separation and, secondly, that those who are committed to the view that all the crucial steps in personality development take place during the first year inevitably have strong motives for calling in question observations pointing to another conclusion. For, if it proves true that grave dislocations of personality development, including deep splits and repressions, can result from experiences that take place in the second and third years (and perhaps also in the fourth, fifth and sixth) and despite satisfactory preceding development, a time-table of personality development such as that proposed by Melanie Klein cannot stand.

The upshot is that such evidence as is at present available points strongly to the likelihood that the processes that underlie detachment are not only defensive in nature but frequently originate during the period of separation itself. A previously impaired development seems in no way a necessary condition for their initiation, though it is likely to be an additional adverse factor. This means that both the first and the third hypotheses are held to be ruled out and the second, that detachment is due to defensive processes which originate during the period of separation itself, is held to stand. As we shall see in the next section, this conclusion is consistent with much analytic theorising including one of the theoretical schemas Freud favoured during his later years.

Loss, a cause of defence: literature

Since, as already remarked, it is not unusual for analysts to contest that defensive processes may be evoked simply by the event of separation, it is of interest to note that, explicitly or implicitly, a number of leading analysts have none the less subscribed to this view. In addition to Anna Freud (in the earlier publication with Dorothy Burlingham & A. Freud, 1942) already quoted, these include Helene Deutsch, Melanie Klein, Fairbairn, and Freud himself. For each of them loss represents a trauma and evokes defence.

In the opening pages of *Studies on Hysteria* (1893–1895) amongst traumas that lead to repression there is listed "the irreparable loss of a loved person" (Freud, 1895d, p.10); and amongst affects that require abreaction are those that give rise to tears. In several of the cases reported on later pages, in which repression and splitting are present, loss and pathological mourning are prominent. From the very first, therefore, loss and grief were recognised by Freud to evoke defence. Nevertheless, although in the last fifteen years of his life the occurrence of repression and splits following loss regains his attention, in the period 1900–1925 there are few references to either.[4] A possible reason for this is that in *Mourning and Melancholia* (Freud, 1917e) the defensive processes following loss are conceived mainly in terms of narcissism and identification. These two concepts not only for some years diverted the attention of Freud but ever since have dominated the thinking on the subject of a majority of analysts.

As a result, it is sometimes overlooked that in the last years of his life Freud once again became concerned with the repression and splits that follow loss. This renewal of interest seems partly to be responsible for and

---

4 [Bowlby notes:] One of the few that by implication refers is his statement in the Introductory Lectures that "there are neuroses which may be described as morbid forms of grief" (Freud, 1916–1917, p.36).

partly to have been encouraged by the reformulation of theory that he undertakes in *Inhibitions, Symptoms and Anxiety*. Towards the end of that work he advanced the view that defensive processes develop to protect the ego from pain (as well as from anxiety) and that a main source of intense pain is loss of loved object. Furthermore, the pain of mourning is to be ascribed, he thinks, to "the high and unsatisfiable cathexis of longing which is concentrated on the object by the bereaved person" (Freud, 1926d, p.172). From this, two conclusions seem logically to follow. The first is that a "high and unsatisfiable cathexis of longing" can evoke defence; the second, that, amongst others, a situation which will inevitably provoke such longing, and therefore defence, is the loss experienced by a young child of his mother. Although Freud came very close to both, in this work he does not seem explicitly to formulate either.

In a paper published only a year later, however, he traces splitting of the ego[5] in the defensive process to a loss sustained in early childhood. In this paper (Freud, 1927) he describes two patients in whom the split had followed loss of father. "In the analysis of two young men", he writes:

> I learnt that each of them – one in his second and the other in his tenth year – had refused to acknowledge the death of his father ... and yet neither of them had developed a psychosis. A very important piece of reality had thus been denied by the ego ...

But, he continues:

> it was only one current of their mental processes that had not acknowledged the father's death; there was another that was fully aware of the fact; the one which was consistent with reality [namely that the father was dead] stood alongside the one which accorded with a wish [that the father should still be living].
>
> (Freud, 1927, p.202)

---

5 [Bowlby notes:] "Splitting of the ego" is the term Freud introduced to denote the state that results when "two mental attitudes have been formed instead of a single one – one, the normal one, which takes account of reality, and another which under the influence of the instincts detaches the ego from reality. The two exist alongside each other" ((Freud, 1938 [1940], p.73). Such a remarkable happening and one so alien to our ideas of the synthetic function of the ego, he suggests, must have its origins in childhood and could hardly occur except "under the influence of psychical trauma" (Freud, 1938 [1940], pp.372–373). (In this last fragment, it should be noted, he illustrates the process by reference to a traumatic experience different from the one with which we are concerned here; it is the discovery that women have no penis).

Although Freud does not relate his discovery of such splits in the ego to the pathology of mourning in general nor to childhood mourning in particular, he did recognise them as the not uncommon sequelae of bereavements sustained in early life. "I suspect", he remarks when discussing his findings "that similar occurrences are by no means rare in childhood". Recent statistical studies show that his suspicion was well-founded.

A similar line of theorising is followed by a number of analysts who have been interested in the clinical problem of patients who are unable to experience grief and some of whom appear indifferent to all human relationships.

A formulation which comes very close both to Freud's and to the one I am advocating is that advanced by Helene Deutsch (1937). In a paper entitled *Absence of Grief* she gives short reports of three patients[6] who, on the one hand, were unable to experience grief and, on the other, frequently suffered from "unmotivated depression". All three shared a similar unfavourable character structure: it took the form of a detachment in relationships with an almost complete lack of emotion. Moreover, they also shared a similar history of loss in childhood. In two cases the patient's mother had died when he was five years old and of each it was said that at the time he had shown no grief; in the other there is no record of early bereavement, but there had been one or more periods of separation in childhood.

From the material obtained in the analysis of the two patients whose mother had died Helene Deutsch advanced two main hypotheses. The first is that the symptoms and the character formation presented are to be understood as the devious expressions of the grief that was not expressed at the time of the childhood loss. The second, which is more tentative, seeks to explain why an individual responds in this way. Although she thinks the condition may occur in an adult as the result of a temporary weakness of the ego following a recent disturbing experience, a main plank in her theorising is that losses sustained in the early years of childhood are specially apt to give rise to it. "The ego of the child is not sufficiently developed to bear the strain of the work of mourning", she suggests:

> It therefore utilises some mechanism of narcissistic self- protection to circumvent the process. If grief should threaten the integrity of the ego, or, in other words, if the ego should be too weak to undertake the elaborate function of mourning, two courses are possible: first, that of

6 [Bowlby notes:] Altogether four cases are reported. Since, however, the character structure of the fourth is different from the other three, that case (No. 4) is omitted from this account. (In an earlier paper (Bowlby, 1962) I have used two of these four cases, Nos. 3 and 4, to illustrate patterns of pathological mourning).

infantile regression expressed as anxiety,[7] and, second, the mobilisation of defence forces intended to protect the ego from anxiety and other psychic dangers. The most extreme expression of this defence mechanism is the omission of affect.

(Deutsch, 1937, p.14)

Since, rightly or wrongly, Helene Deutsch is confident that in at least one of her two patients the previous relationship had been affectionate and undisturbed, she does not hold that a fault in the patient's previous development is a condition necessary for the onset of the defence mechanism. On the contrary, she attributes it simply to an immaturity of the ego in a child of five. (Throughout she speaks simply of a "defence mechanism" and does not discuss its nature).

The psychopathology of her third patient, whose mother had died after he was grown up, Helene Deutsch accounts for rather differently: in him the failure to respond to loss with grief is attributed to the "interference of the aggressive impulse". Scrutiny of the case material, however, suggests that the psychopathology conforms to that of the other two cases more closely than Helene Deutsch supposes.

In his childhood this patient had suffered a temporary separation from his mother[8] and this experience, we are told, had given rise to "intense hate for the mother" with subsequent excessive dependence upon her (a sequence that we now know to be common). When many years later the mother died the old scar, it seemed to the analyst, reopened "The hate impulses which had arisen in a similar situation of disappointment in his childhood were revived" and, instead of grief, he experienced "a feeling of coldness and indifference". Although Helene Deutsch believes this feeling to have been "due to the interference of the aggressive impulse", our increased knowledge of the defensive processes that are evoked by loss in childhood suggests that this may be too limited a view. What seems more likely is that during the childhood separation not only had intense hatred of the mother been aroused but the experience had continued long enough for the small boy to have progressed to the phase Robertson and I have described as detachment, which is of course nothing less than lack of affect for an object lost. On this view, therefore, the absence of grief at his mother's death in later years was due not only to the revival of hate but to the revival also of whatever defence mechanism gives rise to the

---

7 [Bowlby notes:] This idea is based on Helene Deutsch's assumption, discussed in an earlier paper (Bowlby, 1960b), that the small child's reaction to separation is one of anxiety and not of grief.

8 [Bowlby notes:] The separation referred to occurred when the patient was eight years old when a new baby was born; his mother was ill and remained in hospital for some weeks. Helene Deutsch believes, however, that there had been previous separations and that perhaps "the repetition of separation trauma was of importance" (personal communication).

state of "detachment". If this conclusion is correct, the psychopathology of this case, like that of the other two, is to be attributed to defensive processes of a pathological kind that originated following a loss sustained in the early years of life.

When we examine the reasoning underlying Helene Deutsch's theory construction we find two main assumptions. The first is that excessive hatred of the lost object following bereavement in adult life is often attributable to a childhood separation experience; the second that the defence mechanism causing lack of affect is particularly apt to become operative when loss is experienced during any of the early years, including the sixth. Although at several points my formulation differs from that of Helene Deutsch, I believe both these assumptions well-based and consistent with such data as we now have on responses of young children to separation from their mothers.[9]

Another analyst who has drawn attention to the fact that defence mechanisms can be evoked by loss is Melanie Klein. In her paper on *Mourning: Its relation to manic and depressive states* (Klein, 1940) she recognises that grief and longing are themselves painful and that there are "methods of defence which are essentially directed against the "pining" for the lost object" (Klein, 1948, p.316). Unfortunately, however, this perception is often obscured by the complexity of the theory within which she conceives such defence. As a result, the clear recognition that loss itself gives rise to anxiety and pain and itself evokes defensive processes is endangered.

Because the concepts of loss and mourning find only a small place in Fairbairn's writings, the relation of his ideas to the psychopathology of loss tends to be obscured. Nevertheless, that loss can itself give rise to repression and splitting (which he regards, I believe rightly, as different aspects of the same process) is an important part of his thinking. This becomes evident when his theory of an internalized "bad" (namely unsatisfying) object[10] as the keystone of psychopathology is examined (Fairbairn, 1944). For, in the first place, a lost object, because unsatisfying and frustrating, is by definition "bad" and, in the second, being "bad", becomes, according

---

9 [Bowlby notes:] In a recent paper Margaret Mahler (1961) takes a position very similar to that of Helene Deutsch. From about six months of age onwards, she contends, loss of love object leads to grief, which she describes as "a basic ego reaction". "Prompt defensive actions against loss" follow. "Mechanisms ... such as substitution, denial and repression, soon take over in various combinations." Such defensive processes lead, she believes, to the children being left with "lesser or greater scar formation" Although her description of a child's grief as "remarkably short-lived" and his mourning as "transient" can be misleading, her basic theoretical position, like that of Helene Deutsch's, is similar to my own (Mahler, 1961, p.342).

10 [Bowlby notes:] Fairbairn points out that the terms "good object" and "bad object" are misleading and that what is really meant is an object that is sought and that proves either satisfying or unsatisfying (Fairbairn, 1952, p.111).

to Fairbairn, internalised and the primal target for repression. In its turn, the presence of a repressed "bad" internal object leads to a splitting off of that part of the ego which is seeking a relationship with it. Thus, in Fairbairn's view what initiates repression and the ego-splits that are consequent upon it is the presence of an unsatisfying object that has been internalised: and it is evident that of all unsatisfying objects a lost object is one of the most unsatisfying. At a more clinical level of theorising, Fairbairn (1943) advances a view regarding the origins of psychopathy and the defences that underlie it similar to one I myself advanced (Bowlby, 1944). The "callousness and indifference to ordinary human relationships" characteristic of the psychopath, he writes, are to be understood as resulting from "a denial of infantile dependence", and the causes of this "denial" are to be related to conditions in infancy "which made it impossible for him to depend with any confidence upon either of his parents".

A main conclusion that follows from this review is that a number of foremost analysts have recognised that the experience of loss is one of the principal antecedents of defence. In the period 1925–1945 Freud, Helene Deutsch, Melanie Klein, Fairbairn and Anna Freud (in her joint publications with Dorothy Burlingham) each, more or less independently attributed the onset of defensive processes to the experience by the young child of loss of (or separation from) his parents. Four of them, Freud, Helene Deutsch, Melanie Klein and Fairbairn, derived the idea from analytic work on adult character disorders, whilst Anna Freud derived it from direct observation of children in the Hampstead Nurseries. The defences specified are, in the case of Freud, splitting of the ego, in the case of Anna Freud, repression, and in the case of Fairbairn, splitting and repression as different facets of a single process; in this regard Helene Deutsch and Melanie Klein do not commit themselves. In view of these notable contributions it seems puzzling that the notion that loss often evokes defence, including such common defences as repression and splitting, should still remain alien to main traditions of psycho-analytical theorising.

A reading of the literature suggests there are several reasons for this state of affairs, one is that, though each of the five analysts named links the defensive processes they describe to loss, only one, Melanie Klein, links them to mourning: as a result repression and splitting are not always recognised as common ingredients of pathological mourning. A second is that several other analysts, besides not linking their ideas on defence to mourning, have also not recognised that some of the traumatic experiences of early years to which they attribute the onset of defensive processes are best conceptualised in terms of loss. Furthermore, some seem reluctant to identify the defences they describe with repression. Analysts who show some or all of these characteristics are Abraham, Winnicott and Edith Jacobson.

In an earlier paper (Bowlby, 1960b, pp.36–38) I described Abraham's (1924) concept of "primal parathymia" as an antecedent of depressive illness and the part in provoking it that he attributes to disappointments and deprivations that occur in the early years. I then quoted three of his clinical examples, in each of which loss of parent or loss of love is evident. Nevertheless, I pointed out, "in these passages Abraham never uses the words grief and mourning; nor is it clear that he recognised that for the young child the experience of losing mother (or of losing her love) is in very truth a bereavement". Instead of treating these experiences as losses that are apt to give rise to mourning of a pathological kind, the concept invoked is of "a severe injury to infantile narcissism". Because this concept leads in another direction, Abraham's theorising about defence takes a course very different from that advocated here.

In grappling with the problems posed by patients with character disorders of the kind described by Helene Deutsch, Winnicott has advanced hypotheses regarding defence not very different from those she advanced. Thus in a number of papers (e.g., 1954, 1955) he refers to the development of a false self, which he sees as "one of *the most successful defence organisations* designed for the protection of the true self's care" when "the environment behaves not well enough" (1955, italics original). (In this context, by environment Winnicott seems to be meaning mother). In the state of false self the person has difficulty in experiencing his feelings of dependency and, though Winnicott does not state it explicitly, seems likely also to be incapable of experiencing grief. Thus he attributes the development of a personality which is indifferent to ordinary human relationships (an indifference which may be of varying degrees of severity) to the experience in childhood of some failure in parent care. Nevertheless, he does not conceive the nature of the experience in terms of loss of mother or loss of love; nor does he relate his concept of "false self" as a defence either to the pathology of mourning or to the process of repression. Yet it is plain that it is within this frame of reference that his findings and hypotheses are most readily linked to those of Freud and other analysts.

The same criticisms apply to Edith Jacobson. From her studies of depressive illness, this analyst has concluded that traumas occurring during the first five years or so of life are apt to set in train defensive processes of a pathological kind. For example, two patients whom she describes, one a man and the other a woman, had each had an experience at the age of three and a half years to which she attributes pathogenic significance; but in neither case is the experience conceived as a loss nor are the responses evoked by it identified as mourning. Nevertheless, when the experience is examined, it is seen that in each case it amounts to a loss of both parents and that the processes arising conform to those of pathological mourning. The following are brief abstracts of the two cases (for the first case see Jacobson, 1943, 1946, and for the second, 1957). On referral, the female patient, Peggy, aged twenty four, was in a state of severe depression with suicidal impulses and depersonalisation. These symptoms had been precipitated by a recent loss, actually the loss of her lover. The childhood experience on which Edith Jacobson places major emphasis occurred when Peggy was three and a half years old. At this time her mother went to hospital to have a new baby, whilst she and her father stayed with the maternal grandmother. Quarrels developed and father departed.

"The child was left alone, disappointed by her father and eagerly awaiting her mother's return. However, when the mother did return it was with the baby". Peggy recalled feeling at this time "This was not my mother, it was a different person", (a feeling that we now know is not uncommon in young children who have been separated from their mothers for a few weeks). It was soon after this, Edith Jacobson believed, that "the little girl broke down in her first deep depression".

During the course of the analysis Peggy suffered many depressions. She would then "feel deserted by both parent representatives", "would indulge in spiteful phantasies of living alone without love", and would also "start long affectionate dialogues with herself, playing a mother soothing and caressing her baby". Summing up, Edith Jacobson describes what she believes the internal processes to be: "In her disappointment and hostility [Peggy] tries to escape into a narcissistic withdrawal. She decides to kill her need for love and to become absolutely self-sufficient and independent".

The male patient (Jacobson, 1957) was in his early thirties and:

> combined a compulsive-depressive personality structure with tendencies to act out and to develop sporadic psychosomatic and hysterical conversion symptoms... . His main complaint [however] was that his emotional life was so dull and subdued. He was a 'detached onlooker'.

In this case the childhood experience to which Edith Jacobson attributes his disabilities was a "trauma that had broken up his relationship to his mother" and which (as in the case of Peggy) had occurred when he was three and a half years old. At this time his mother had had a miscarriage. His father was absent and, although his mother remained at home, she "had been physically sick and depressed for many weeks after... . Left in the hands of a maid, he had felt lost and confused".

Thenceforward, it appears, he had shown either "cold resentment" towards his mother or "cold detachment" from her. During the analysis, however, there were evoked in him "waves of affection towards his mother", which hitherto had been repressed.

Now it may be questioned both whether the happenings in these patients' early childhoods were accurately recalled and also whether Edith Jacobson was right in attributing to them so much significance for her patient's emotional development. But, if we accept, as I am inclined to do, both the validity of the events and their significance,[11] I believe the concept of loss to be the one best fitted to describe the experience, and that of pathological mourning the one best fitted to describe the responses to which in each case it gave rise. The way that each patient is said to have responded to the loss of mother with repression of love and yearning, resulting in detachment from her and from others, is particularly striking. In her discussion, however, the author utilises neither of these concepts. Instead, following the lead of Abraham, she uses concepts such as "disappointment" and "disillusionment" and "narcissistic injury", which have a different significance and are not easily related to mourning. A representative passage runs as follows: "Early disappointment must therefore have the effect of a narcissistic injury in consequence of and along with the devaluation of the disappointing object of love" (Jacobson, 1946, p.132).

Thus, a main reason for the slow recognition of childhood loss as a cause of repression and splitting seems to be that the link has not been made between, on the one hand, childhood trauma and defences of repression and splitting to which all recognise it gives rise and, on the other, childhood loss and processes of pathological mourning which follow it. There is, however, another and perhaps weightier reason. This is the strong tradition in analytic theory construction which, by emphasising fixation in the oral phase and/or a phase of primary narcissism as the major determinant of depressive illness, has led to the belief that the events of most consequence for the development of a capacity to mourn occur in the first year of life. Since, as already noted, empirical evidence does not seem to support this view, it is desirable, first, to examine the grounds on which it is held and, secondly, to consider whether an alternative hypothesis can be framed able to embrace both the traditional data derived from the treatment of patients and the new data derived from observations of how young children respond to loss of a love object.

Six characteristics of depression[12]

Extreme sadness is a dominant feature of depressive illness. Extreme sadness, either unbroken or in spasms, is a prominent feature also of young children away from their mothers; indeed were it not so frequently underestimated it would hardly need emphasis. Moreover such sadness resembles closely the sadness of adult mourning, especially in its yearning for the object lost and in refusal of substitutes.

---

11 [Bowlby notes:] In the case of Peggy there is reason to believe that the separation at three and a half was only the culmination in a series of disturbances in her relation to her mother, who is described as a dominating woman who disciplined the child severely.
12 [Editors' note:] Subtitle missing from the text. Added by the editors.

A second major feature of depressive illness which is also characteristic of young children away from their mothers is an absence of organised activity and a loss of interest in the environment. Let me repeat parts of Robertson's description of such a child given in an earlier paper: "During the phase of *Despair* ... the active physical movements diminish or come to an end. ... He is withdrawn and inactive [and] makes no demands on the environment" (Bowlby, 1960a, p.90).

A third feature common to patients suffering from depressive illness and to young children separated from mother is some deviation of oral behaviour; though, apart from transitory refusal to eat, the disturbance seen in young children is, in contrast to depressive adults, more often an excess of activity than a reduction of it. For example, Dorothy Burlingham and Anna Freud (Burlingham & A. Freud, 1942, 1944) refer not only to the intensity and prolongation of thumb-sucking in the Nursery children but also to their "insatiable greed"; both forms of behaviour, they state, are due to "sudden separation from the mother". Amongst the examples they quote is the case of Tom:

> About the age of two years, he lost contact with his mother who abruptly ceased her visits to him. He became extremely dissatisfied and developed three rather disturbing reactions; violent thumb-sucking; over-eating; and passionate temporary attachments to strangers and guest-workers.
>
> (Burlingham & A. Freud, 1944, p.60)

The strong tendency of young children in hospital or residential nursery to eat far more than they do at home has also been recorded by Robertson. In addition, he has observed how, when they remain away for long periods, their interest in their parents is often replaced by intense preoccupation with food.[13]

A fourth feature of depressive illness is the tendency of patients to displace towards themselves reproaches and hostile acts which would more appropriately be directed towards a lost object. Although, as Engel (1962) has pointed out, less common as a symptom than sadness and inactivity, this feature is the one that as much as any has been responsible for the classical psycho-analytical theories of melancholia. What evidence, we may therefore ask, is there that this tendency also is encouraged by loss in childhood? There is in fact a great deal, and once again relevant observations have been recorded both by Dorothy Burlingham and Anna Freud and by Spitz. Furthermore, each has explicitly drawn the conclusion that

---

13 [Bowlby notes:] Elsewhere (Bowlby, 1960c) I have discussed some of the possible processes by which such behaviour might be brought about.

when a young child suffers loss and deprivation, aggression is particularly apt to be directed against the subject himself.

Dorothy Burlingham and Anna Freud discuss the theme in connection with head-banging which, they observe, appeared in the Nurseries at about the age of one year. Because "it is usually accompanied by crying," they continue:

> one might be led to believe that the child cries as a result of the pain inflicted on it by knocking or banging its head. But closer observation shows that it is rather the other way round. The child first cries as an outlet for its anger and frustration and then follows up this expression with the more violent one of head-knocking ... [it] is a sign of ... impotent anger.
>
> (Burlingham & A. Freud, 1944, p.60)

Spitz (1953, pp.126–138) describes different though related behaviour in an infant of eight months. This infant:

> after prolonged separation from its mother, would violently hit the left side of its face with its fist by the hour in a rhythm comparable to head banging. This child directed the blows always at the same spot on the left side of its face under certain specific circumstances which aroused its resentment. The blows were well co-ordinated.

From this observation and others, he had made, Spitz, concludes, tentatively, that "the deprived infant's aggression, which cannot be directed against an outer world object, is returned against the self". In drawing this conclusion, he is supported by what he has observed happens after the infant's return to his mother. The infant then "no longer hits or scratches itself. It now begins to bite, to scratch, to kick *others*" (Spitz, 1953, italics in the original).

Another form of behaviour, which is probably also related to the expression of aggression towards the subject himself, has been recorded by Robertson (Robertson, 1953b). This is the propensity of young children in hospital or residential nursery to destroy their own toys. For example, he records how one small girl of two years and nine months who was back in hospital for a second time soon after a five-week stay was given by her mother a so-called indestructible doll. Not only had this little girl within a week destroyed the doll but each time the ward sister effected repair she systematically repeated the performance.

By just what processes behaviour of this kind is brought about is difficult to know. As Cain (1961) in a valuable review of the problem has pointed out, there is no reason to suppose that, for aggression to be "turned-inward", a complex differentiation of psychic structure is necessary. Self-attack, he notes, is not uncommon in captive primates; the examples he quotes show, moreover, that it is apt to be provoked when the animal loses either the human experimenter or the company of another animal it likes. Nevertheless, even if theory remains in debate, the facts are reasonably assured. From the second half of the first year onward (and possibly before) loss of mother not infrequently leads the child to injure itself.

Thus, when four main features of depressive illness – extreme sadness, inactivity and loss of interest, orality and self-attack – are considered, each is found to be frequent, indeed characteristic, of young children after they have lost their mothers. In addition, two features in the personalities of those prone to the illness – the tendency to make ambivalent relationships and to show narcissistic behaviour – are characteristic also of children who, having lost mother, are now either reunited with her or else have become partially attached to a substitute. Let us consider each successively.

Of the many features of depressive illness none has been so universally remarked upon by analysts as the disposition of its victims between attacks to show intense ambivalence in their object relations, namely both intensified demand for the object and intensified hatred when demands are not met. Now, apart from constant threats by a parent not to love him or to go away and leave him, no experience to which a young child is likely to be subjected is better calculated to intensify his ambivalence than one or more periods away from his mother in strange hands. Both intense clinging and following and also intense anger when for any reason he is prevented from doing so, usually expressed in a temper tantrum,[14] are found to be practically universal on return home.

Finally, by initiating defensive processes, a period of separation from mother can exacerbate or produce all those phenomena that have traditionally been attributed to narcissism, namely a difficulty in making object relations, and especially of maintaining them in conditions of frustration or disappointment, and excessive preoccupation with self, including auto-erotism. Many examples of such behaviour in the Hampstead Nurseries are described by Dorothy Burlingham and Anna Freud (Burlingham & A. Freud, 1944). The theoretical proposition to which these observations point, namely that narcissism can readily be understood as secondary to frustration of object relations, is argued strongly by Balint (1937) and Fairbairn (1952) and is an integral part also of my position.

This completes our review of six salient features of depressive illness and of personalities prone to it, about which there is unanimity of opinion and to explain which all psychoanalytic theories aspire, and demonstrates that each one of them occurs regularly, or at least frequently, in young children who have

---

14 [Bowlby notes:] A useful way to conceptualise the affect which a depressed patient is unable to express is, I believe, as a temper-tantrum directed against a deserting object.

lost their mother, either fairly recently or longer ago. This finding, taken with our knowledge, such as it is, of the childhood histories of depressed patients, gives strong support to the hypothesis that it is in experiences of loss, actual or threatened, occurring not only in the first year but in the succeeding ones also, that the vital roots of at least some forms of depressive illness are to be found. This is a revised version of Abraham's hypothesis of primal parathymia.

Plainly the account of the hypothesis as given is no more than an outline and to be adequate would need much further development. It would need, for instance, to be encompassed within a broader theory of depressive illness which takes account not only of other types of unfavourable experience in the early years besides loss, temporary or permanent, or threat of loss, but also of genetic factors. The purpose of this enquiry, however, is not to explain depressive illness but to explore the effects of losses occurring in the early years. The reason for this rather long excursion into the theory of depressive illness is, indeed, no more than to clear the ground of what I believe to be an unfounded assumption – that events of the first year of life are the main determinants of pathological mourning and, therefore, the main determinants also of the defences that underlie it.

One strength of the theoretical position I am advocating is, I believe, that it enables a theory of pathological mourning to be related readily to a theory of pathological anxiety.

Pathological mourning and pathological anxiety

The very close relationship of pathological depression to pathological anxiety has long been recognised. So too has the connection of both with, on the one hand, grief and separation anxiety and, on the other, guilt and intensely ambivalent object relationships. No theory that is unable to explain these inter-connections is satisfactory.

The theory advanced here takes as its starting point Freud's conception that anxiety is a reaction to the danger of loss and the pain of mourning a reaction to actual loss. To this it adds –

1. that loss and threat of loss always give rise to intensified ambivalence towards the object and so, by processes which Melanie Klein has made familiar, to both a further increase of anxiety and to an increase of guilt.
2. that loss itself can, at least in the early years, give rise to defensive processes of pathological degree and so to the development of object relationships of the kind often termed narcissistic.

From this it follows that, when loss is sustained or repeatedly threatened in early childhood, the individual is often rendered prone to make intensely ambivalent and narcissistic relationships, to suffer excessive anxiety and guilt, and to respond to later loss by pathological mourning.

The theory is in keeping with our knowledge both of the responses of young children to loss and also of events that are common in the childhood histories of those who later develop pathological anxiety and pathological mourning. It is, moreover, susceptible to test at a number of points.

Conclusion

In this paper it has been shown that study of the empirical evidence regarding detachment as it occurs in young children removed from their mothers suggests strongly not only that detachment is due to defensive processes but also that these processes have their origin during the period of separation itself. Although not widely recognised to be so, this conclusion is consistent with much of Freud's thinking about defence. Theories that hold that in children of over one year such defensive processes occur only in those whose development is already impaired are shown to be hardly consistent with data; they derive from reconstructions of infant development that are hypothetical and at many points open to question.

Several questions arise from this conclusion. One is concerned with the period of life during which loss can evoke defensive processes in persons hitherto mentally healthy. In this study the fact that it can do so in children during their second and third years has been emphasised because it is to this age-group that our observations refer. There seems no reason to doubt, however, that it can do so as well both in younger and in older subjects, namely during the first year of life and also after the third birthday. It may be, indeed, that in some degree defensive processes can be evoked by losses sustained at almost any age. However, that may be, it is losses that occur during the early years of life, especially the first five or six, that seem especially apt to have pathological consequences.

Nevertheless, not all individuals who are exposed to situations of loss in the early years develop disturbed personalities, and those that do so suffer disturbance of very varying form and degree. If such variations are not to be attributed wholly, or even mainly, to the path that development has taken prior to the loss, it may be asked, to what variables are they to be attributed? Those that I believe will repay systematic investigation are the ones that operate at the time of the loss and after it. Such variables are not only very numerous but differ according to whether the loss is temporary or permanent (Ainsworth & Bowlby, 1954). Amongst others, they include those relating to the immediate circumstances of the loss, those relating to substitute figures, for example their familiarity or otherwise and their continuity or otherwise, those relating to the degree to which the child's feelings and strivings are understood and responded to, for example during a separation by substitute figures and after it by his own mother, and those relating to repetition of loss. To what extent differences of outcome can be traced to the effects of these and similar variables is at present unknown. Only, however, when the assumption, common in psychoanalytic circles, that all differences are due to the state or stage of development by the child at the time of the loss is abandoned will the necessary research be undertaken. My strongest plea, therefore, is that the question be recognised as open.

The main conclusion of this paper, namely that experiences of separation in the early years readily give rise to defensive processes, forms an integral part of the set of hypotheses I am advancing regarding the conditions that determine the onset, in the years beyond childhood, of pathological variants of mourning and so of much psychiatric illness. It is one, moreover, that in addition to practical implications, raises a number of issues in the theory of defence. A study of the defences that follow loss becomes, indeed, a study of many of the fundamental problems of defence.

References

Abraham, K. (1924). A short study of the development of the libido, viewed in the light of mental disorders. In: K. Abraham (Ed.), *Selected Papers on Psycho-Analysis*, (1927) (pp. 418–501). London: Hogarth Press.

Ainsworth, M. (1967). *Infancy in Uganda*. Baltimore: The Johns Hopkins Press.

Ainsworth, M. D. & Bowlby, J. (1954). Research strategy in the study of mother-child separation. *Courrier de la Centre International de l'Enfance*, 4: 105–131.

Balint, M. (1937). Early developmental states of the ego. Primary object love. In: M. Balint (Ed.), *Primary Love & Psycho-Analytic Technique* (pp. 90–108). London: Hogarth Press.

Bowlby, J. (1944). Forty-four juvenile thieves: Their characters and home life. *The International Journal of Psycho-Analysis*, 25: 19–53.

Bowlby, J. (1954). Some psychopathological processes set in train by early mother-child separation. In: M. J. N. Senn (Ed.), *Problems of Infancy and Childhood* (pp. 38–90). (Proceedings of the 7th May, 1953, Josiah Macy Jr. Foundation Conference on Infancy and Childhood. New York: Josiah Macy Foundation.

Bowlby, J. (1960a). Separation anxiety. *The International Journal of Psycho-Analysis*, 41: 89–113.

Bowlby, J. (1960b). Grief and mourning in infancy and early childhood. *Psychoanalytic Study of the Child*, 15: 9–52.

Bowlby, J. (1960c). Ethology and the development of object relations. *The International Journal of Psycho-Analysis*, 41: 313–317.

Bowlby, J. (1961). Separation anxiety: A critical review of the literature. *Journal of Child Psychology & Psychiatry*, 1: 251–269.

Bowlby, J. (1962). Pathological mourning and childhood mourning. *Journal of the American Psychoanalytic Association*, 11: 500–541.

Bowlby, J. & Robertson, J. (1956). A two-year-old goes to hospital. In: K. Soddy (Ed.), *Mental Health and Infant Development. Vol.1: Papers and Discussions*, pp. 123–124. London: Routledge and Kegan Paul.

Burlingham, D. & Freud, A. (1942). *Young Children in Wartime.* London: Allen & Unwin.

Burlingham, D. & Freud, A. (1944). *Infants Without Families.* London: Allen & Unwin.

Cain, A. C. (1961). The presuperego 'turning-inward' of aggression. *The Psychoanalytic Quarterly, 30*: 171–208.

Deutsch, H. (1919). A two-year-old boy's first love comes to grief. In: L. Jessner & E. Pavenstedt (Eds.), *Dynamics of Psychopathology in Childhood* (pp. 1–9). New York: Grune Stratton.

Deutsch, H. (1937). Absence of grief. *The Psychoanalytic Quarterly, 6*: 12–22.

Engel, G. L. (1962). Anxiety and depression-withdrawal: The primary affects of unpleasure. *The International Journal of Psycho-Analysis, 43*: 89–97.

Fairbairn, W. D. (1943). The war neuroses – their nature and significance. In: W. D. Fairbairn (Ed.), (1952) *Psychoanalytic Studies of the Personality* (pp. 256–288). London: Tavistock Publications.

Fairbairn, W. D. (1944). Endopsychic structure considered in terms of object relationships. *The International Journal of Psycho-Analysis, 25*: 70–92.

Fairbairn, W. D. (1952). *Psychoanalytic Studies of the Personality.* London: Tavistock Publications.

Freud, A. (1960). A discussion of Dr. John Bowlby's paper "Grief and mourning in infancy and early childhood". *Psychoanalytic Study of the Child, 15*: 53–62.

Freud, S. (1893a). *The Psychical Mechanism of Hysterical Phenomena.* [with J. Breuer]. *S. E., 2*: 3–17. London: Hogarth Press.

Freud, S. (1895d). *Studies on Hysteria.* [with J. Breuer]. *S. E., 2.* London: Hogarth Press.

Freud, S. (1915d). *Repression. S. E., 14:* 143–158. London: Hogarth Press.

Freud, S. (1916–1917). *Introductory Lectures on Psycho-Analysis. 1916–1917. S. E., 15–16.* London: Hogarth Press.

Freud, S. (1917e). *Mourning and Melancholia. S. E., 14*: 239–258. London: Hogarth Press.

Freud, S. (1925h). *Negation. S. E., 19*: 235–239. London: Hogarth Press.

Freud, S. (1926d). *Inhibitions, Symptoms and Anxiety. S. E., 20*: 77–174. London: Hogarth Press.

Freud, S. (1927 [1940]). Fetishism. In: *Collected Papers of Sigmund Freud* (pp. 198–204). London: Hogarth Press.

Freud, S. (1938 [1940]). Splitting of the ego in the process of defence. In: *Collected Papers of Sigmund Freud* (pp. 372–375). London: Hogarth Press.

Freud, S. (1940). *An Outline of Psycho-Analysis.* London: Hogarth Press.

Heinicke, C. M. (1956). Some effects of separating two-year-old children from their parents: A comparative study. *Human Relations, 9*: 105–176.

Heinicke, C. M. & Westheimer, I. (1961). *Brief Separations.* London: Longmans.

Hinsie, L. E. & Shatsky, J. (1940). *Psychiatric Dictionary.* London: Oxford University Press.

Jacobson, E. (1943). The Oedipus conflict in the development of depressive mechanisms. *Psychoanalytic Quarterly, 12*: 541–560.

Jacobson, E. (1946). The effect of disappointment on ego and superego formation in normal and depressive development. *Psychoanalytic Review, 33*: 129–147.

Jacobson, E. (1957). Denial and repression. *Journal of the American Psychoanalytic Association, 5*: 61–92.

Klein, M. (1940). Mourning and its relation to manic-depressive states. In: M. Klein (Ed.), *Contributions to Psycho-Analysis* (pp. 311–338). London: Hogarth Press.

Klein, M. (1948). *Contributions to Psycho-Analysis*. London: Hogarth Press.

Lindemann, E. (1944). The symptomatology and management of acute grief. *American Journal of Psychiatry, 101*: 141–148.

Mahler, M. E. (1961). On sadness and grief in infancy and childhood. *The Psychoanalytic Study of the Child, 16*: 332–335.

Rado, S. (1928). The problem of melancholia. *The International Journal of Psychoanalysis, 9*: 420–438.

Robertson, J. (1953a). Film: *A Two-year-old Goes to Hospital*. London: Tavistock Child Development Research Unit.

Robertson, J. (1953b April). Some responses of young children to the loss of maternal care. *Nursing Times*, 382–386.

Robertson, J. & Bowlby, J. (1952). Some responses of young children to separation from their mothers. *Courrier de la Centre International de l'Enfance, 2*: 131–142.

Spitz, R. A. (1953). Aggression. Its role in the establishment of object relations. In: R. M. Loewenstein (Ed.), *Drives, Affects, and Behavior* (pp. 126–138). New York: International University Press.

Winnicott, D. W. (1954). Mind and its relation to the psyche-soma. *British Journal of Medical Psychology, 27*, 201–209.

Winnicott, D. W. (1955). Metapsychological and clinical aspects of regression within the psychoanalytical set-up. *International Journal of Psychoanalysis, 36*, 16–26.

Appendix

A letter from Mary Ainsworth to John Bowlby commenting on this paper,
Loss, Detachment and Defence
   [Editors: Wellcome Trust Library Archive PP/Bow/D.3/69–70]

7511 Club Road,
Ruxton, 4, Md.,
Dec. 11, 1962

Dr. John Bowlby
Tavistock Clinic
Beaumont Street
London, W.1.

Dear John,
When I was in the army I learned that each separate topic should have
a separate memorandum or letter, so that each could be filed neatly in its
own special file. This letter is going to abuse that useful rule, for I have
many topics in mind.

First, may I congratulate you on *Loss, Detachment and Defence.* It seems to
me to round off the series for your book *The Psychopathology of Loss* much
better than the previous version. I cannot comment in detail on the improve-
ments because Jim Deese has my copy of the earlier version. In general, however, I think it is wise of you to omit your general discussion of motivation,
for that is bound to be very controversial – and before you could have coped
with all that arose from the controversy you would have had to add two or
more chapters and another year or so!
   I read through the paper carefully, in the hope I might be helpfully critical,
but apart from a few picayune details which were probably typographical
errors and will certainly be picked up, I had only one major comment –
centering on your discussion of the difference between your term "detachment" and Anna Freud's term "withdrawal." But, as I read it over again
I realized that Anna Freud's term "withdrawal" was both descriptive of
behavior and of underlying process (withdrawal of cathexis) while "detachment" you use to describe behavior and go on to specify the processes of
repression, denial and splitting. It is still a little confusing to the reader.
Even I made a marginal protest that "detachment" and "withdrawal"
weren't all *that* different. So I think, in your subsequent argument, and not

merely on page 8, you could replace the word "detachment" at least sometimes by "detached behavior" just to help keep people straight.

I became curious enough about these terms to look them up in "Webster's Dictionary of Synonyms." I am sure you have done something, of the same sort, and given terminology much more thought than I have, but just in case you have not hit on this particular source I quote bits – which I feel support your position on the whole.

"Detached" – synonyms - aloof, disinterested, indifferent, unconcerned, incurious.

"Detach" – "one detaches something when one breaks (literally or figuratively) a connection, a tie, or a bond, and thereby isolates it or makes it independent."

"Detached" – "in comparison with indifferent, aloof etc. (less fortunately) often implies a commendable aloofness which is the result of freedom from prejudices or of selfish concern for one's personal interests."

"Withdraw" – synonyms - remove or draw.

"Withdraw" – "implies a taking back or away someone or something that has been placed elsewhere."

It seems to me clearly that Anna Freud is using the right word to say what *she* means, and you are using the right word to say what *you* mean – on the behavioral level – for it certainly appears from behavior that the child's tie with the mother has been broken.

My other general comment is totally uncritical. It is merely that your argument in the paper as a whole rings true to me.

Where do you stand now? Is the one book all but completed? And where do you and Jimmy stand in regard to the other?[15]

Second, I have been receiving some very gratifying feedback from the published results of my frantic year of writing. Re the WHO paper, which has really scarcely gotten out here, I have had some very good responses. Two of the people whose opinion I most respect are Harry Harlow and Julius Richmond who were very enthusiastic and are using the paper in teaching. Moreover the whole issue (i.e. the WHO Health Paper) is going to be reviewed for *Contemporary Psychology* by Leon Yarrow, and so it will scarcely be "buried" as far as the American psychologists are concerned. Meanwhile, I have been asked to review a review by Yarrow for the new Annual Review of Child Development Research (I think the title is), so at

---

15 [Editors' note:] Ainsworth is referring to an unpublished book manuscript that was the object of repeated revisions from the mid-1950s to mid-1960s. The book reported research findings from the study of hospitalised children. Bowlby, J., & Robertson, J. *Protest, Despair and Detachment*, PP/BOW/D.3/38

least we can be polite to each other! Meanwhile the other sequelae are coming – invitations to participate in symposia and the like.

The as yet unpublished paper on African babies I sent to John Whiting of Harvard, who wrote back that it was not only the best study on the Baganda he had seen but one of the best on any non-literate society. (I don't know why I still need this kind of approbation, but it is a shot in the arm to forge ahead with the larger publication.)[16]

The four Acculturation papers with Len as co-author have not received as much attention, but this I don't mind for all I cared about was discharging a duty in a scientifically respectable way. Nevertheless, they have served to reopen warm professional interaction with my former colleagues at the EAISR in Kampala, most of whom are people I value.

Third, I report progress on the book on the Baganda babies and their mothers. I have not progressed as quickly as I had hoped, but I suppose that's inevitable. But I have it about two-thirds written – and the worst part is over. The new editor of the Johns Hopkins Press expresses the same interest in it as did his predecessor. We have arranged to have typed and circulated among more readers what I have done so far. (I am having it dittoed rather than typed, so I can circulate it to people whose opinions I value regardless of whom the Press chooses as official readers. And you would certainly be one of these.) The notion is that one whole revision may be saved by circulating it at this stage of development.

As I told you, I intended to write it in a way suitable for a variety of readers – those anthropologists and cross-cultural psychologists interested in methods of child rearing; child development people in several formal disciplines; and also perhaps the intelligent layman interested in Africa, babies, or perhaps only in his fellow humans. In this effort I may have erred. Perhaps I have made it too chatty and personal for the tastes of the scientists, and still failed to make it of interest to the so-called Intelligent layman. Perhaps it is too detailed – and I am a very bad judge of that for I am inclined to be too wordy and besides I find all these details of Baganda life in general and of my sample in particular so fascinating that it is difficult for me to imagine that other people wouldn't find them equally interesting. Should there be more or less case material? And that general sort of thing is what concerns me at this stage. I would be most grateful to have your opinion – directly or through JHU Press or both – and hope that the first segment will be in the mail by the first of the year.

---

16 [Editors' note:] The "larger work" would eventually be: Ainsworth, M. (1967). *Infancy in Uganda*. Baltimore: The Johns Hopkins Press.

My new project,[17] by the way, has been deferred until I get an advanced draft of the African book completed. I can imagine tidying and revising whilst beginning a new project, but not the main writing task. Needless to say, I feel guilty, for the grant began Oct. 1st. But I guess this sort of thing has happened before.

Fourth, you may be interested to know that I was asked to organize a symposium for the meeting of the Society for Research in Child Development in Berkeley in April. Bettye Caldwell and Harry Harlow are joining me in co-ordinated papers on "Longitudinal Studies in Infant–Mother Interaction." Among other things I hope thereby to give a plug to short-term longitudinal studies which are in bad repute in this country just because long-term longitudinal studies have proved unmanageable.

Finally, I come to a point that is really none of my business for I am not a Member of the Tavistock Study Group. But even as a guest I feel enough identified with it to make suggestions. I have two suggestions as to people you might be interested in including in the next meeting.

1. Bettye Caldwell. who is doing longitudinal research in mother–infant interaction at the Upstate Medical Center of the State University of New York. My contacts with her have not been close to date, but I have heard her speak and read her papers. She strikes me as a very happy combination of the warm, personal Myriam David sort of person, the sophisticated psychologist who knows the methods and the issues, and, to top it off, a psychologist who is both "au fait" and balanced in her interest in and knowledge of the animal behavior field.

I am a little disappointed that her own research is being conducted in the well-baby clinic based on observations of interaction there rather than in homes, but it looks good for all that it is not in the home setting. The home is best if one can get there.

2. Daniel Lehrman, of whom you may well have heard, but who came into my ken just recently. He is a comparative physiological psychologist who seems to me to combine three disciplines most expertly— psychology, physiology and ethology. He spoke at a JHU Psychology Symposium, and gave one of the best talks of its sort I have ever heard, impressing one as a sensitive observer, an excellent experimenter and a most entertaining speaker. He spoke on reproductive cycles in ringdoves, reporting a most ingenious and productive series of experiments that enabled him to demonstrate the intimate interaction between interpersonal (inter-bird) interaction,

---

17 [Editors' note:] Likely the Baltimore longitudinal study home observations.

behavior and physiological (hormonal chiefly) processes, both in heterosexual and parent–child relations. I asked for reprints, and my opinion of him is not lessened by the written word – although I have not read all of it. I know that Harlow has a high opinion of both Caldwell and Lehrman. As far as Lehrman is concerned, you would want Robert Hinde's opinion, but I can't imagine that they would not respect each other. Lehrman and Rosenblatt seem be close, and I gather that Lehrman is considered more highly than Rosenblatt. There, I have said my piece about these two, and it is up to you and the situation. I will say no more.

This letter has gone on long enough. As you can gather things are going well with me – and I thank you for your encouragement that helped make them go well.

With best personal regards,
As ever

Mary Ainsworth

Chapter 3

The place of defensive exclusion in depressive disorders

[Editors: c.1978–1979. Chapter written for, but not included in, Bowlby's book *Loss*. Wellcome Collection Archive PP/BOW/K.7/94]

Cognitive disconnection of response from eliciting event

Already in this volume (*Loss,* Bowlby, 1980), e.g. in Chapters 13, 22 and 23, there are references to the tendency for adults and children whose mourning is taking a pathological course to be unclear or even wholly ignorant of what it is that is making them depressed. It is therefore in keeping with expectations that this same tendency has been noted repeatedly by analysts studying the psychology of depressive disorder.

A very early reference to the phenomenon is to be found in Freud's *Mourning and Melancholia* in which he expresses the suspicion that a melancholic patient:

> cannot consciously perceive what he has lost … This would suggest that melancholia is in some way related to an object loss which is withdrawn from consciousness, in contradistinction to mourning in which there is nothing about the loss that is unconscious.
>
> (Freud, 1917e, p.245)

Other and more explicit references to the disconnection of response from recent events are to be found in several systematic studies of depressive disorders, for example those of Cohen et al. (1954), of Beck (1967), of Sachar and others (1967), and of Weissman and Paykel (1974), as well as in many of the less systematic ones.

Among twelve patients diagnosed as suffering from manic-depressive psychosis studied by Cohen & her colleagues (1954) was a man whose psychotherapist wrote:

> the outstanding therapeutic problem … was that of getting the patient to think in terms of 'psychic causality'; that is, to recognize there was

a connection between what he experienced in his dealings with others and the way he felt. He was unable to recognize, for instance, that when someone did something to slight him, this would lead to his having hurt feelings.

(Cohen, 1954, p.129)

In illustration the therapist describes how a little before Christmas the patient, who had recently begun some part-time teaching, complained during his session of not feeling well. He then reviewed events of the preceding days and in amongst things referred briefly to the fact that, like other members of the faculty, he had received a present from the students. Only by a chance question from the therapist, however, was the upsetting nature of that experience revealed. Whereas some of the more senior teachers had received rather magnificent presents, he, the newcomer, had received little more than a token. Only then, when recounting the story, did he become aware of how hurt by this he had felt.

In similar vein, Beck (1967) refers to patients who "may pass through several depressive episodes without identifying the pairing of the depression with a recurrent set of traumatic conditions", and he also gives an example.

Sachar's study of brief psychotherapy

One of the most systematic studies yet done on the part played by what I am terming disconnection of response from eliciting event in patients suffering from depressive disorders was undertaken by Edward Sachar, a psychiatrist and psychoanalyst then working at Harvard (Sachar et al., 1967, 1968). In this sophisticated study Sachar's aim was to test the hypothesis, derived from psychoanalytic thinking, that in depressive disorders many of the typical symptoms operate so as "to help the patient *avoid* experiencing the painful loss" and, in particular, enable him to avoid considering both the meaning that the loss has for him and its implications.

In designing his project Sachar's reasoning was as follows: When psychotherapy is guided by the hypothesis stated, a principal part of the therapeutic task is seen as that of helping the patient confront the loss and its implication, or, to put it into the language introduced in Chapter 4, (Bowlby, 1980) to help him accept for processing information that, although registered by him in a preliminary way, had henceforward been defensively excluded. From this it can be predicted that, during the time that the patient is engaged on the task, he will be in a state of much greater emotional distress than he will be either before doing so or afterwards. One way of testing whether that is so or not, Sachar noted, would be by making use of certain endocrinological findings of Hamburg's

(1962), which had shown that during states of emotional distress the excretion rate of adrenal corticosteroids increases.

In the light of that, Sachar predicted, the excretion rates of these steroids would increase during the confrontation phase of psychotherapy and would decrease again when the task was completed.

To test these predictions Sachar and his colleagues studied six women who had presented with depressive symptoms. Selection was based on the following six criteria:

(a) the disorder was of recent onset and appeared to be reactive to a clearly defined event
(b) the patient's condition required her admission to hospital
(c) schizophrenic features were absent, both in the symptomatology and in the previous personality
(d) signs of a medical illness also were absent
(e) the patient had received neither ECT nor hormone therapy during the previous year
(f) the patient appeared suitable for short term psychotherapy in regard to both basic personality and intelligence.

As regards provoking events, although in all cases they are classified by Sachar as losses in only one was it a death. One patient had had a quarrel with her mother, who had been critical of her. Another had lost her girl friend. A third, a teacher, had found herself unable to maintain discipline. A fourth had lost her husband by death. A fifth, a widow living with her daughter, had discovered her daughter was having an affair; and the husband of the sixth was instituting divorce proceedings after fourteen years of marriage.

During their stay in hospital two classes of data were collected and kept wholly independent. One class comprised the measurement over each 24 hour period of the amount of certain corticosteroids excreted in the patient's urine. The other class comprised data about the patient's psychological state, for which the procedure was as follows.

After admission a detailed history was obtained from each patient by a resident or a social worker, and psychological tests (Rorschach & The Minnesota Multiphasic Personality Inventory, MMPI) were given. Throughout the patient's stay the nurses kept daily notes. Twice weekly each patient received analytically oriented psychotherapy in which, in Sachar's words, "the emphasis [was] on confronting and resolving the precipitating depressive issue, that is, the loss and its meaning to the patient". Sessions were taped. In addition, after each session a summary of the topics dealt with was dictated, together with the therapist's impression of any critical events and his description of the patient's appearance, affect state, manner of speech and way of relating.

After the patient's discharge and without knowledge of the endocrine findings Sachar and his colleagues met in conference to review the psychosocial data and, by consensus, to designate when they believed the confrontation phase of psychotherapy to have begun and when it had ended. This phase they defined as the period of psychotherapy during which "the loss and associated fantasies appeared in consciousness with a vividness and a graphic detail such that there was imparted a quality of reliving the painful events", and during which affect appropriate to the events was expressed and the behaviour and thought patterns hitherto characteristic of the depressive disorder were disrupted. The phase was judged to have ended when the patient's depressive symptoms had abated and she was able to plan her future fairly realistically.

When, for each patient, the levels of steroid excretion for the days designated as those of confrontation were compared with the levels of excretion during the days before and after, the levels measured during confrontation were found to be significantly higher for five of the six patients. Thus, with one exception (which the authors discuss), the initial prediction was confirmed.

Although in his discussion of these results Sachar sometimes uses a more traditional language than the one I am using, the theory behind his thinking is almost the same as mine. Several conclusions can be drawn from this clinical experiment. In each of the five patients who followed the predicted pattern there is reason to believe that during an initial phase, termed by Sachar the phase of depressive equilibrium, information about an event of much emotional importance was being defensively excluded, with the result that little or no processing of its meaning could take place and, as a further consequence, no affect of relevance was aroused. Instead of such further processing and of the affect that would have been aroused by it, moreover, the patient's mind was occupied by a variety of thoughts which, although of a disagreeable nature, had little or no connection with the provoking event. These ruminating depressive thoughts, together with whatever behaviour goes with them, Sachar regards as defensive operations, namely operations which serve to divert the patient's attention away from thinking about the event and its implications.

Support for this formulation comes from the consequences of the therapist's efforts to help the patient consider in honest detail the nature of the event that had provoked her depression, what had led up to it, and what its implications for her might be. Once started on this process, not only did each patient think differently but she also felt differently. In Sachar's words:

> The quality and intensity of experienced affect also changed, to an emotional state consisting of mixtures of sadness and anxiety, best described in terms such as anguish, grief, desperation and helplessness;

the release of anger was also a feature in three cases. These affects seemed somehow more human and moving than those seen during the depressive equilibrium phase, and invited empathetic responses from staff members.

(Sachar, et al. 1968)

During this phase, moreover, patients began to see the person lost in a more realistic light and "also became more aware of and involved with therapeutic figures at this time".

With the six depressive patients the results were uneven. Three patients recovered, one recovered partially but was thought not to have dealt fully with her problem, a fifth recovered partially but relapsed, and the sixth, who had had a previous psychotic depression ten years earlier, "was overwhelmed by the experience and required ECT, following which she recovered". There follows here a summary of one of the patients who did well.[1]

Mrs EE was thirty four years old, divorced with two children. On admission she suffered severe headaches and fatigue, criticised herself for being a bad mother, and felt her past to be worthless and her future hopeless. She made strong demands on the ward staff and consoled herself with ideas that they would transform her from an unlovable ugly duckling into a lovable swan. Prior to admission she had experienced impulses to get drunk, to become promiscuous and to hurt herself or her children.

The events judged to have provoked her condition had taken place during a period of a few weeks when her mother had stayed at her house. The mother (described by the authors as "narcissistic and psychopathic") had borrowed a large sum of money from Mrs EE., had entertained a man she had picked up, had castigated her daughter for not being nice to him, and had accused her of being a bad daughter. Despite this treatment, Mrs EE., when questioned, said little against her mother. Asked if she had been disappointed, she replied "Well I expected a little more"; and on another occasion remarked "After all, she's all I've got."

In formulating their hypothesis about how the provoking event had affected Mrs EE, the clinicians concerned invoke the concept of loss: "In the view of the workshop the patient had experienced the loss primarily as an injury to her basic sense of being lovable, with associated latent feelings of abandonment, and intolerable rage at being betrayed."

The confrontation phase of therapy began on day twenty seven, just prior to which Mrs EE had begun to recall many painful experiences of childhood, including abandonment and rejection by her mother.

1 [Bowlby notes:] This account, rewritten, is taken from Sachar & others (1968).

On that day Mrs EE had also been asked to take a job in the hospital. This led to a strong outburst against the staff, described in the original account as follows:

> 'You don't care about me', she cried. 'You are treating me just like my mother.' 'I know you will throw me out if I disobey you', she wept, 'but something inside of me cries 'No''. As the staff held firm, the patient's despair deepened; she got drunk one night and threatened suicide on another. At the same time many relevant early memories of rejection by mother and grandmother were recalled.... The therapist and administrator were finally able to clarify for [her] the difference between present and past, and her distortion of the present situation in the light of earlier experiences.

Following this phase, which lasted ten days, Mrs EE felt that the staff respected her after all:

> She said in wonderment, 'I have a right to get angry', a right she began to exercise appropriately with the staff. Her spirits lifted, many of her depressive symptoms disappeared, her self-esteem rose, and she was able to accept limits and a realistic job.

In keeping with the clinician's predictions corticosteroid levels were higher during three of the ten days of confrontation than on any day either before or afterwards.

Comment

Though I see this patient's problems from a perspective very close to Sachar's, my formulation of them is a little different. First, in his formulation the term loss is used ambiguously and in a way I find confusing. An alternative formulation would be that, despite her mother having abused Mrs EE's hospitality and having simultaneously dubbed her a bad daughter, Mrs EE was unable to construe her mother's behaviour towards her as unfavourably as others might do and her own role as more sinned against than sinning. Instead, she accepts her mother's picture of her – that she is a bad daughter and a bad mother. Instead, therefore, of feeling angry with her mother she feels angry with herself; and instead of directing murderous feelings towards her mother, she directs them towards herself and her children. This mode of construing their relationships she maintains during the phase of depressive equilibrium, by excluding defensively all memories of how cruelly her mother had treated her in the past (probably also by dwelling on her own misdeeds).

One reason why Mrs EE felt constrained always to see her mother in a favourable light and herself in an unfavourable one can be inferred from

Mrs EE's assumption that if she disobeyed the hospital staff she would be thrown out. Whenever as a child Mrs EE had felt tempted to disobey her mother or criticise her, this leads me to infer, her mother had threatened to abandon her and may, indeed, actually have done so on occasion.

In the case report the events that had preceded Mrs EE's breakdown are given in only the barest outline, which leads me to wonder what the context was of the various disagreements she had had with her mother? A conjecture that goes only a little beyond what is given is that during these weeks any move by Mrs EE to criticise her mother had been met by her mother not only accusing her of being a bad and unlovable daughter but once again threatening to have nothing further to do with her.

Thus, instead of the situation experienced by this patient being seen, in Sachar's words, "as an injury to her basic sense of being loveable", I see it as one in which Mrs EE was feeling not only unloveable but in imminent danger of being abandoned.

References

Beck, A. T. (1967). *Depression: Clinical, Experimental and Theoretical Aspects.* London: Staples Press.

Bowlby, J. (1980). *Attachment and Loss: Volume III: Loss, Sadness and Depression.* London: Hogarth Press.

Cohen, M. B., Baker, G., Cohen, R. A., Fromm-Reichmann, F., & Weigert, E. (1954). An Intensive Study of Twelve Cases of Manicdepressive Psychosis. *Psychiatry, 17*: 103–137.

Freud, S. (1917e). *Mourning and Melancholia. S.E., 14*: 239–258. London: Hogarth Press.

Hamburg, D. A. (1962). Plasma and urinary corticosteroid levels in naturally occurring psychological stresses. In: S. R. Korey, A. Pope, & E. Robins (Eds.), *Ultrastructure and Metabolism of the Nervous System* (pp. 169–181). Baltimore: Williams and Wilkins.

Sachar, E. J., Mackenzie, J. M., Binstock, W. A., & Mack, J. E. (1967). Corticosteroid responses to the psychotherapy of reactive depressions. I. Elevations during confrontation of loss. *Archive of General Psychiatry, 16*: 461–470.

Sachar, E. J., Mackenzie, J. M., Binstock, W. A., & Mack, J. E. (1968). Corticosteroid responses to the psychotherapy of reactive depressions. II. Further clinical and physiological implications. *Psychosomatic Medicine, 30*: 23–44.

Weissman, M. M. & Paykel, E. S. (1974). *The Depressed Woman: A Study of Social Relationships.* Chicago: University of Chicago Press.

Chapter 4

Darwin

Psychiatry and developmental psychology

Contribution to a Symposium on Darwin and Psychology held at the Conference of the British Psychological Society, London, December 1983.
[Editors: Wellcome Collection Archive PP/BOW/F.3/132]

A major influence of the Darwinian revolution has been to emphasize the presence of continuities in natural phenomena where formerly only dichotomies had been seen. In some fields this shift in perspective has for long been complete, or as complete as such shifts ever are: Man is an animal species and not in a realm of his own; the races of mankind are not separate species but variants of a single one. But in other fields the shift has been very slow and even a century after Darwin's death is still controversial. My aims in this paper are twofold. One is to give an account of how the influence of this shift has been and still is affecting two disciplines in which Darwin took an interest – developmental psychology and psychiatry. The other is to show how the belated introduction into these disciplines of Darwinian principles is enabling heartening progress to be made.

In the field of psychiatry Janet Browne (1985) has already described how the practitioners of Darwin's day, thinking in terms of discrete categories of mental disease, were bent on identifying facial expressions diagnostic of each category and how Darwin could see nothing of the kind. To his fresh untutored eye the photographs sent him portrayed distressed human beings exhibiting, often in intense degree, the ordinary human emotions of rage, fear and sorrow. In the present day this conflict of viewpoint is still with us.[1] The categorists are still searching for diagnostic criteria that distinguish the mentally ill from the normal, though today their search is more likely to be for genetically determined biochemical anomalies than

---

1 [Editors' note:] The landmark third edition of the American Psychiatric Association Diagnostic and Statistical Manual of Mental Disorders (DSM-III) had been published in February 1983, to great fanfare. The DSM-III is widely recognised as a key moment in the rise to dominance of diagnosis-based psychological practice.

for any behavioural criterion. Those others who, like myself, believe continuity to be a more fruitful perspective point to the steadily increasing evidence of the part played by exposure to certain types of disturbed family interactions during infancy, childhood and adolescence in accounting for differing degrees of vulnerability to emotional disturbance and mental breakdown. The respective advantages in psychiatry of these different perspectives are still to be determined.

The immense influence exerted by Freud in both psychiatry and psychology has been mainly to emphasize continuities. Again and again he expressed the desire to develop a psychology capable of embracing healthy as well as pathological psychic functioning, a psychology in which the pathological appears as merely a distorted version of the normal; and he also strove ceaselessly to establish continuities in socio-emotional development from states of early childhood into adult life.

In this ambitious programme Freud made progress; yet his was no more than a beginning and one unfortunately that proved difficult to build upon. The comparative stasis in psychoanalytic thinking that has been all too evident since Freud's death nearly half a century ago can be traced, I believe, to his having failed to grasp the strength's of Darwin's approach to problems of adaptation and evolution and having instead based his theory on biological principles now long discredited. Thus, as Frank Sulloway (1979) has shown, Freud drew on Haeckel's Law of Recapitulation in order to sketch his picture of child development, which it must be remembered had no empirical foundation, and he drew on some of Lamarck's least useful ideas when considering problems of adaptation and motivation. As a result of these false moves during a sensitive phase of its development, psychoanalysis is only now starting to replace Freud's theory of libidinal phases with an empirically based theory of socio-emotional development, and is still stranded without any agreed theory of motivation: whilst Freud's theory of psychic energy has few friends, there is still no sign of agreement on what should take its place.

Darwin's study of the emotions

The aim of Darwin's study of the emotions in man and animals was as a test of his thesis that man has evolved as a species within the animal kingdom. The forms in which the various emotions are expressed in different species of mammal, especially in the primates including Man, are sufficiently alike, he suspected, as to indicate some degree of biological affinity. This would imply, amongst much else, that the emotions and their expression in Man are in some degree genetically pre-programmed (to use modern terminology). In order to test this hypothesis Darwin collected data from many fields. One field was other countries and cultures. Do members of other cultures show the same facial expressions and gestures as Western Europeans?

When someone is surprised, for example, does he show the same facial appearance and gestures no matter what his country, race or culture? Another field, as we have already heard, was mental hospitals. A third field was infants in whom, he believed, it might be possible to observe "the pure and simple source" from which our expressions spring. Whereas for several fields he had to rely mainly or wholly on the observations of correspondents, the observations of infants could be his own.

As early as 1840 after his first child, William, was born Darwin began making observations of the expressions of emotion in human infants. Many of these observations are recorded and discussed in his book on *The Expression of the Emotions in Man and Animals* (1872). The record of his observations on William appeared five years later under the title *A Biographical Sketch of An Infant* in the journal *Mind* (1877).

In collecting his data Darwin relied on the systematic observing and recording of behaviour as it occurs in the natural setting. In the course of his sketch of William, he describes at least seven common emotional states each of which is accompanied by a distinctive facial expression. Most of these states he describes in considerable detail, with constant reference to the contraction of particular facial muscles. By the time his son had reached fifteen and a half months he had observed and described all of the following: anger, fear, affection, pleasure, amusement, discomfort and jealousy; and during subsequent months he recorded shame, embarrassment, grief and resignation.

Darwin discusses many of the methodological problems that arise in such a study. For example, some expressive movements are ambiguous and make it difficult to infer the infant's state of mind. Knowledge of the stimulus situation can bias observation. Darwin was suitably cautious. In making his inferences he took into account the whole response. A flushed face can suggest a number of emotions; but when accompanied by bright eyes, compressed mouth and clutched fists inference is restricted.

Not only did he observe during the early months of infant life expressions characteristic of the various emotions in forms similar to those seen in adults, but his observations also led him to conclude that "An infant understands to a certain extent, and as I believe at a very early period, the meaning or feelings of those who tend him, by expression of their features" (Darwin, 1877, p.294).

From these observations, as well as those gleaned from other fields he explored, Darwin concluded that in humans there is continuity both of emotional expression and of understanding across ages and across cultures, and continuity in some degree also across species. Human expressive behaviours are the products of Man's evolution and are therefore biologically determined characters.

Since Darwin reached that conclusion much water has flowed under the psychological bridges. For a time radical behaviorism seemed to many to have relegated Darwin's views to a prejudiced past. The mind of an infant, it was held, is little more than a tabula rasa on to which information is writ by means of learning and from which it is expunged by means of extinction. Not everyone subscribed to that view; but for three-quarters of a century empirical research on emotional expression was conspicuous by its absence.

How then stands the field today?

Recent research on the emotions

The short answer is simple. Research during the past two decades on the expression of the emotions during infancy and childhood and in peoples of many different races and cultures, most of it stimulated by Silvan Tomkins (1962, 1963), has uniformly supported Darwin's conclusions. Ten years ago in a valuable volume edited by Paul Eckman (1973), compiled to celebrate the centenary of Darwin's book, Charlesworth and Kreutzer (1973) review Darwin's observations of infants in the light of studies then recently conducted and that used far more rigorous methodology. Their conclusion was that up to that time, whilst Darwin's observations had been amply confirmed, "surprisingly little" had been added. Since those words were written, however, much more detailed observations have been made using modern video technology and much new has been discovered. Precursors of different emotional expressions as well as germinal recognition of the emotional expressions of others can be reliably observed, it is found, considerably earlier than formerly reported. Because affects are only fleetingly expressed during the early days and weeks of life, to obtain valid results it is necessary to engage in prolonged spells of observation.

Let me give a few examples.

Colwyn Trevarthen in Edinburgh has been one of the pioneers in the current resurgence of research. Having noticed that by the age of two months an infant is showing a pronounced difference in his responses to persons and to inanimate objects, he has designed a situation in which a mother can engage in face-to-face social interaction with her infant whilst, by means of a mirror, a ciné camera is able to take pictures which record the facial expressions of both infant and mother on the same frame. Using these techniques he has been able, during the second month of life, to demonstrate "the wide range of moods and emotions, pre-speech and gestures, obviously preformed for conversational communication and animated signalling". The expressions of infants two-to-three months old, he reports, "are organized in episodes of a few seconds in length that resemble sentences. They are interpreted by mothers as 'speaking'," and lead to lively interchange in which there is impressively close co-ordination between the responses of the two partners. As a result of these studies Trevarthen concludes that "emotional states should be defined within personal interaction rather than as supposed moods of an isolated individual" (Trevarthen, 1979).

Comparable studies in the United States have led to similar conclusions. For example, in his study of Jenny, an abused and neglected child of just under four months, Thomas Gaensbauer (1982) emphasizes how transient emotional expressions are during early life, but also how flexible, prompt and situationally specific they are, especially to different people. Although the expression of emotion is usually extremely brief, such expressive episodes tend to be repeated. This implies an underlying emotional state of which the changes in facial expression are but intermittent indicators.

Using the detailed criteria for identifying each of the common facial expressions that have been described by Caroll Izard (1982),[2] Gaensbauer (1982) reports how at four months Jenny showed the following emotions: sadness, fear, anger, interest, and enjoyment. Each was associated with some other typical behaviour and was elicited by very specific situations. For example, when her face showed fear Jenny withdrew bodily, averted her eyes and turned towards her mother. This she did when approached by a male but not by a female: the physical abuse had been from father not mother. Similarly, an expression of interest-curiosity was accompanied by increased animation and attention to environment, and she also leaned forward. These patterns occurred when she was interacting with a female stranger but only when no male was present.

The hypothesis that patterns of facial expression are pre-programmed, as all these studies suggest, is further supported by the finding that they occur in blind-born children, who are observed to laugh, smile, sulk, cry, and to show surprise and anger. Furthermore, the same motor patterns are seen in members of every culture yet studied (e.g. Eibl-Eibesfeldt, 1972).

This is not to say that learning plays no part. For example, blind children express emotion less frequently and less intensely than sighted children. In one culture the expression of an emotion may be confined to certain narrowly defined situations whereas in another may be seen in response to a much wider range of comparable situations.

Within any one culture, moreover, the frequency and intensity with which different individuals show each of the principal emotions are found to differ greatly and, certainly in children, to be correlated with the way their parents treat them. Thus, not surprisingly, infants with happier experiences than Jenny's are likely to show the positive emotions of interest, joy and surprise much more frequently than she did. Now that researchers have available methods for identifying the different emotions, longitudinal studies are showing that at least during the first four or five years of life one of the most stable characteristics of individual children is the balance of the emotion that they show when exposed to different everyday situations (Sroufe, 1983).

2 [Bowlby notes:] For references to his earlier publications see Izard (1982).

Not only are mothers well able to recognize the different emotions expressed by their infants and to respond adaptively to each, but it is confirmed too that, as Darwin suspected, babies a few moths old are well capable of discriminating the expression of an adult's face. Indeed, experiment shows that even neonates can discriminate between three affective facial expressions – a smiling face, a surprised one and a sad one – by responding distinctively to each (Field & Walden, 1982, reported by Demos, 1982).

Thus, after a long period of eclipse, developmental psychology has now not only recovered the position in which Darwin left it a century ago but is at least progressing well beyond it. The human infant is seen as born preadapted to participate in social interchanges by means of emotional communications and to be genetically biased to develop co-operative social relationships provided his maternal partner plays a reasonably helpful part. This image of infancy is a far cry from the images long presented to students by academics and clinicians alike.

Implications for psychiatry and psychoanalysis

The shift in perspective I am describing is due in great part, of course, to the influence of ethology which, a direct descendant of Darwin's studies of behaviour and firmly based on Darwinian principles, is for the first time providing the behavioural sciences with a solid biological foundation. Among the many advantages that ethology has brought is that it is now possible to reformulate psychoanalysis in such a way that it can be integrated into the main bodies of psychology and psychiatry and of the other biological sciences instead of existing in a private world of its own.

A great deal of psychoanalysis is concerned to understand and to help individuals who find themselves either chronically anxious or depressed or else incapable of loving and perhaps also filled with anger. Although Freud's original model of the mind was that of an isolated system designed to reduce stimulation, as clinical experience was gained it became evident that the disturbances of emotional life from which patients suffer are best understood as aspects of disturbed personal relationships. This recognition led to the development in Britain of the object-relations school of psychoanalysis, identified with the names of Melanie Klein, Ronald Fairbairn and Donald Winnicott, and in the United States of the neo-Freudian school, linked to the names of Erich Fromm, Karen Horney and Harry Stack Sullivan. Although I believe these were major steps forward, they nonetheless resulted in a bewildering array of overlapping and competing theories, some very complex and speculative, and with no agreed means for selecting among them. The term "object" in object relations, moreover, a left over from Freud's early theorizing, is singularly ill-suited to refer to the image of a live human being with whom the individual has for long interacted.

Among many key issues about which there has been controversy are how to understand behaviour traditionally termed dependency, anxiety about separation, and the relation between depression and loss. These are all matters with which I became concerned some years ago whilst engaged in trying to explain the intense distress shown by a young child when he finds himself in a strange place with strange people and his tendency to respond with acute anxiety to any sign that such an experience might be repeated. The first task, I concluded, was to understand the nature of the child's tie to his mother.

At that time, in the early fifties, there was no agreement on how to account for this. The dominant theory, advanced by Freud and widely held, was that a child becomes interested in his mother because she feeds him. Two kinds of drive are postulated, primary and secondary. Food is thought of as primary; the personal relationship, referred to as dependency, as secondary. This theory did not seem to me to fit the facts. For example, were it true, an infant of a year or two should take readily to whomever feeds him and this clearly was not the case. An alternative theory, advanced by Melanie Klein (1948), was also closely linked to food, and was again a secondary drive theory of personal relations. Variations in development were then attributed by her to events occurring during the earliest months and limited to the feeding relationship, with much emphasis on breasts and orality. Once again I thought the theory failed to fit the facts: variations in development seemed to be influenced far more by the mother's general attitude toward her child and how she treats him than by what happens simply during his feeding.

Yet, if the prevailing theories were inadequate, what were the alternatives?

That was when I first heard of ethology and the experiments of Lorenz on the following responses of goslings who develop a tie with mother without the intermediary of food. This provided an alternative model that had a number of features that seemed possibly to fit the human case. After due reflection on our data, it seemed reasonable to advance the hypothesis that the human infant comes into the world genetically biased to develop a set of behaviour patterns that, given an appropriate environment, will result in his keeping more or less close proximity to whoever cares for him; and, further, that this tendency to maintain proximity serves the function of protecting the mobile infant and growing child from a number of dangers, amongst which in man's environment of evolutionary adaptedness the danger of predation is likely to have been paramount. The various forms of behaviour that serve to maintain a child in proximity to his mother could then conveniently be grouped together under the term attachment behaviour (Bowlby, 1958, 1969).

From this standpoint it became possible to see separation anxiety in a new light. Why "mere separation" should cause anxiety had for long been a mystery. Freud wrestled with the problem and advanced a number of hypotheses (Freud, 1926d). Every other leading analyst has done the same. With no means of evaluating them, many divergent schools of thought have proliferated and much fruitless debate been engendered.

The problem lies, I believe, in an unexamined assumption, made not only by psychoanalysts but by more traditional psychiatrists as well, that fear is aroused in a mentally healthy person only in situations that everyone would perceive as intrinsically painful or dangerous, or that are perceived so by a person only because of his having become conditioned to them. Since fear of separation and loss does not fit this formula, analysts have concluded that what is feared is really some other situation; whilst traditionally minded psychiatrists have supposed that the patient's anxiety must derive from some biochemical or endocrine derangement.

The difficulties disappear, however, when an ethological approach is adopted. For it then becomes evident that man, like other animals, responds with fear to certain situations, not because they carry a *high* risk of pain or danger, but because they signal an *increase* of risk. Thus, just as animals of many species, including man, are disposed to respond with fear to sudden movement or a marked change in level of sound or light because to do so has survival value, so are many species, including man, disposed to respond to separation from a potentially caregiving figure and for the same reasons. Once seen in this perspective, the problem is solved (Bowlby, 1973).

Loss gives rise to grief and mourning, a field for long of central concern to psychoanalysts but, once again, one about which there has been no agreement. It happens, however, that these are problems to the understanding of which Darwin himself made important contributions which, when rediscovered and applied, have proved of the greatest clinical value.

The facial expressions of adult grief, Darwin concluded (1872), are a resultant, on the one hand, of a tendency to scream like a child when he feels abandoned and, on the other, of an inhibition of such screaming. Both crying and screaming are, of course, means by which a child commonly attracts and recovers his missing mother. They occur in adult grief, it is found, as part of the same motivation, namely an urge to recover the person lost. This urge, which may be conscious or unconscious, is now well recognized, and knowledge of its presence has helped to explain many of the more puzzling features both of healthy and of disordered mourning (Bowlby, 1961; Parkes, 1969). It has also helped demonstrate that the mourning responses of children and of adults lie on a continuum, yet another matter about which there has been prolonged disagreement (Bowlby, 1980).

This is not the occasion to pursue these ideas further. Suffice it to say that by adopting an ethological approach it has proved possible to construct a new conceptual framework within which the clinical data of psychoanalysis – the real core of the discipline – can, I believe, be understood and examined afresh. In this new framework distinctions between causation and function and current ideas regarding instinctive behaviour, adaptation, and the role of environment, all play central roles. Among its merits is the impetus to empirical research, both developmental and clinical, to which it has given rise.

References

American Psychiatric Association. (1983). *Diagnostic and Statistical Manual of Mental Disorders* (DSM-III). Washington, DC: American Psychiatric Association.

Bowlby, J. (1958). The nature of the child's tie to his mother. *The International Journal of Psycho-Analysis, 39*: 1–23.

Bowlby, J. (1961). Processes of mourning. *The International Journal of Psycho-Analysis, 42*: 317–340.

Bowlby, J. (1969). *Attachment and Loss: Volume I: Attachment*. London: Hogarth Press.

Bowlby, J. (1973). *Attachment and Loss: Volume II: Separation, Anxiety and Anger*. London: Hogarth Press.

Bowlby, J. (1980). *Attachment and Loss: Volume III: Loss, Sadness and Depression*. London: Hogarth Press.

Browne, J. (1985). Darwin and the face of madness. In: W. F. Bynum, R. Porter, & M. Shepherd (Eds.), *The Anatomy of Madness: Essays in the History of Psychiatry, (Vol. 1), People and Ideas* (pp. 151–165). London: Tavistock Publications.

Charlesworth, W. R. & Kreutzer, M. A. (1973). Facial expressions in infants and children. In: P. Ekman (Ed.), *Darwin and Facial Expressions: A Century of Research in Review* (pp. 91–168). New York, NY: Academic Press.

Darwin, C. R. (1872). *The Expression of the Emotions in Man and Animals*. London: John Murray.

Darwin, C. R. (1877). A biographical sketch of an infant. *Mind: A Quarterly Review of Psychology and Philosophy, 2*: 285–294.

Demos, V. (1982). Affect in early infancy: Physiology or psychology. *Psychoanalytic Inquiry, 1*: 533–574.

Eckman, P. (1973). *Darwin and Facial Expression: A Century of Research in Review*. Cambridge, MA: Malor Books.

Eibl-Eibesfeldt, E. (1972). *Love and Hate: The Natural History of Behavior Patterns*. New York: Holt, Rinehart, & Winston.

Field, T. & Walden, T. (1982). Production and perception of facial expressions in infancy and early childhood. In: H. Reese, & L. Lipsitt (Eds.), *Advances in Child Development and Behavior* (Vol. *16*, pp. 169–211). New York: Academic Press.

Freud, S. (1926d). *Inhibitions. Symptoms and Anxiety. S.E., 20*: 77–174. London: Hogarth Press.

Gaensbauer, T. J. (1982). The differentiation of discrete affects: A case report. *Psychoanalytic Study of the Child, 37*: 29–66.

Izard, C. (Ed.) (1982). *Measuring Emotions in Infants and Children*. Cambridge: Cambridge University Press.

Klein, M. (1948). *Contributions to Psycho-Analysis*, 1921–1945. London: Hogarth Press.

Parkes, C. M. (1969). Separation anxiety: An aspect of the search for a lost object. In: M. H. Lader (Ed.), *Studies of Anxiety* (pp. 87–92). (British Journal of

Psychiatry Special Publication No. 3.). London: World Psychiatric Association and the Royal Medico-Psychological Association.

Sroufe, L. A. (1983). Infant-caregiver attachment and patterns of adaptation in preschool: The roots of maladaptation and competence. In: M. Perlmutter (Ed.), *Minnesota Symposium in Child Psychology* (Vol. 16, pp. 41–83). Hillsdale, NJ: Erlbaum Associates.

Sulloway, F. (1979). *Freud, Biologist of the Mind: Beyond the Psychoanalytic Legend.* New York: Basic Books.

Tomkins, S. S. (1962). *Affect Imagery Consciousness: (Volume I), The Positive Affects.* London: Tavistock.

Tomkins, S. S. (1963). *Affect Imagery Consciousness: (Volume II), The Negative Affects.* London: Tavistock.

Trevarthen, C. B. (1979). Communication and cooperation in early infancy: A description of primary intersubjectivity. In: M. Bullowa (Ed.), *Before Speech: The Beginning of Interpersonal Communication* (pp. 321–348). Cambridge: Cambridge University Press.

Part 2

Early writings on guilt, anxiety, and identification

Chapter 5

Psychological problems of evacuation

[Editors: c.1939–1942. Wellcome Collection Archive PP/BOW/C.5/4/1]

Those whose normal peace-time work take them into daily contact with the psychological problems of family life, difficult children and foster homes are surprised not at the breakdown of evacuation but at its partial success. For if there is one thing which experience of medical psychology and child guidance work impresses upon one it is the immense emotional importance of home and family life. Unfortunately the ill effects of bad homes have received far more attention than the good effects of the normal home. Indeed some amateur enthusiasts have drawn the conclusion that modern psychology thinks children are better brought up away from their homes. This is the equivalent to saying that because bad food gives us indigestion we should be wiser to eat nothing.

The truth is that every human being from birth to old age draws emotional sustenance and strength from those few people who constitute his home. Love and friendship are as vital to man, especially the child, as bread and coal.

These simple human needs need restating in a world preoccupied by economic stress and political strife. They need restating also because they are the essential background against which the emotional problems of the evacuation must be seen. For the evacuation has broken up family life all over the country.

Adolescents 11–16 years

The normal adolescent has often been very homesick when in strange quarters, but there is little evidence of deeper emotional disturbances. Much of this homesickness has been cured by visits either of child to parent or of parent to child. The few occasions when visits have ended badly seem to have obscured the generally beneficial effects of visits. All workers in touch with the children testify to this.

The explanation lies in the reassurance which children get that their homes and parents are safe and well and they themselves are welcomed and loved. Such worries have been extremely common and usually unvoiced. The fear that London has been bombed and their homes destroyed is after all not surprising when the expectation of this was the very reason for their having left. Such anxieties about the well-being of home and family are normal to childhood in the same way that they are normal in an absent father or mother. The well-balanced child can deal with such anxieties but some of the less stable have collapsed.

Another frequent cause of adolescents being unsettled has been their impatience to leave school. This naturally has affected the 14 and 15 year olds who have felt that they were profiting little from the sketchy education provided and felt they would be better off at work.

Children of 6 to 10 years

Adolescents have a certain amount of self-confidence and independence in the world. Their estimation of themselves is not entirely dependent on what others think of them. To some extent they can laugh at the irritable die-hard or the fussy maiden lady. But younger children have fewer resources of their own. They are largely at the mercy of public opinion especially the opinion of their parents or foster-parents. To be in good odour is to be happy – to be in bad odour is to feel unwanted and unsafe. Few children go through this period without days when they feel no one loves them or being haunted by fantastic fears of being turned out of hearth and home for being naughty and disobedient. Such fears are normal but fortunately in the average home there is constant reassurance against them.

But when a small child is sent to a foster-home things may be very different. In the first place he *has* been sent away from home. It is true that it has been for his safety but not all children can believe the truth. The child who feels unwanted, whether this is really so or only his imagination, will find it very difficult not to interpret his being sent away as his parents' desire to be rid of him. In Child Guidance work one finds this belief again and again in children who have been sent to hospital or a foster-home. Often it is only half-expressed or half-believed. But it is just as real a fear as the fear of bogey-men in the dark – also only half-believed and perhaps less than half-admitted. This fear is behind the great unhappiness which a few small children have suffered during the evacuation. Such emotional experiences whether justified by his mother's attitude or the result entirely of imagination and misinterpretation may leave a child miserable and insecure, bearing a grudge against his parents and society in general for a long while to come. Thus the result is exactly contrary to what many people suppose. The child who feels happy and safe in his own home is the child who settles best in a foster-home. It is the child who has felt unhappy and insecure at home who finds it most difficult to leave it.

The fear of not being wanted will vary very much with the emotional conditions in a child's home and it will be only a minority of children who are seriously affected. None the less quite normal children may feel it to some extent and this together with anxiety over the safety of parents and friends was one of the principal causes of the outbreak of bedwetting in the early days of the evacuation. There seems general agreement that about three-quarters of the cases of bedwetting occurred in children who were in no sense chronic bedwetters. The emotional upset of leaving home, the strangeness of new people, fears of doing the wrong thing, in a few cases a cool reception, all these make a child feel awkward and uneasy. When we add to these troubles makeshift beds and strange sorts of lavatory it is not surprising that many children lost control of their bladders.

Those with experience of children recognised that much of the bedwetting was transitory and knew how best to handle the problem. One woman experienced in handling problem children took in ten bedwetters who had been turned out of other billets and by making them feel at home, keeping them warm in bed and making it easy for them to get out during the night had eight of them dry within a week. The other two turned out to have been chronic bedwetters prior to evacuation. Although in almost every case where the condition was serious investigation showed it to have existed long before the evacuation.

In all cases of emotional disturbance the important factor is the child's feelings about being reft away from home and mother and his fear that for one reason or another he will never see either again. It is natural therefore that those children who have been made to feel most at home in their new surroundings should have suffered least. Where foster-parents have welcomed the children and made them feel that they were liked and wanted, most children have been fairly happy. Some of the most unsuccessful cases have been where children have been taken in to a big house and made to live with the servants. The servants have not always treated them very kindly and they have felt homeless and unwanted. Moreover almost all cases where a dozen or more children have been billeted *en masse* in a big house have been failures, except where a genuine home atmosphere has been created. The children have become wild disobedient little hooligans, an attitude quickly changed where they have been re-billeted with a number of homely foster parents. It is for these reasons that psychological opinion does not favour camps, at any rate for children under eleven. The recent popular vote on this subject was something of a red-herring. For the public knows the admitted disadvantage of foster-homes, but has no knowledge whatever of the disadvantages of camps which experience may easily prove to be far greater.

Infants and toddlers

Perhaps in no sphere of the evacuation have the effects of ignorance and wishful-thinking been more apparent than in the enthusiasm shown in some quarters for the whole-sale evacuation of the day-nurseries and nursery schools to which toddlers normally go for a few hours each day whilst their mothers work. For when small children are separated from home and given for long periods to the care of strangers in strange surroundings their whole character development may be seriously endangered.

Anyone who has had a child of his own will have realised the extreme dependence and attachment which small children have for their mothers and the one or two other women whom they are used to. In spite of this the belief is prevalent that because a child is small it does not matter who looks after him provided he is kindly treated. Certainly it is remarkable how happy small children can often appear when looked after by strangers. But there is now a great deal of evidence that this happiness is deceptive. Small children when in the hands of strangers for long periods, especially when these strangers come and go, become more and more emotionally isolated until in some cases they cease to be able to become attached to anyone at all. It is a slow insidious process, so slow and insidious in fact that its progress may not be recognised until the severe emotional damage has been done.

Research into the origins of persistent delinquency in childhood has recently thrown this question into high relief. The majority of child delinquents are probably normal children up to mischief. But they of course are not the serious problem. The serious problem is the chronic and persistent delinquent who pilfers anything he can lay his hands on, lies inconsequently, truants, wanders and has no social sense. Now in a large number of these cases the child's bad character can be traced unequivocally to prolonged separation from his mother (or mother substitute) in early childhood. Some have been in hospital for long periods, others in a succession of foster-homes, in others again mother has been ill and the baby has been in a hostel. The one common factor however is separation from the people who are known and being looked after by complete strangers in strange surroundings for long periods – six months or more. For instance in a recent research undertaken at the London Child Guidance Clinic the records of forty-four juvenile thieves were studied. Of the forty-four, thirty-one proved to be children who had stolen regularly and repeatedly. Of these thirty one serious cases no less than seventeen had been away from their homes with strangers for six months or longer during their first five years of life. This high proportion contrasts with only three of a control group of forty four problem children who did not steal. Despite the small sample the difference is statistically significant. (Incidentally other researches have indicated that in the general population only about 1% of children have suffered such a separation.) *The conclusion is that the prolonged separation of small children from their homes is one of the outstanding causes of the development of a criminal character.*

No scheme for the evacuation of young children which ignores this fact should be considered. Meanwhile we should bear in mind that there are at present many thousands of young children who have been placed unwittingly in circumstances gravely jeopardising their future. Not only are some likely to develop into criminal characters as a result of their experiences but many others may be expected to become prone to chronic anxiety or depression or to vague pains and illness of an apparently physical nature. The semi-delinquent character who is grasping, jealous and not above much petty cheating may also follow.

It is important to remember the parents of these children. The mothers of small children who have been evacuated for long periods alone will at the end of hostilities find themselves greeting home children who do not know them, who regret leaving their foster-parents or nurses, who will be resentful and disobedient children and remain difficult or delinquent characters. If these facts are squarely faced it will be seen that provision for the safety of the under fives is an immensely grave and difficult problem.

The parents of evacuated children

Very little consideration has been given to the parents of the children who have been evacuated. What references there have been have been almost universally disparaging. They have not kept the children clean or trained them properly, they upset the children by their visits, they invade the foster-homes on Sunday, above all they are wicked and selfish either not to send the children away or else to bring them home again.

But let us consider the question from the parents' point of view. Are they really so bad and perverse as they are made out?

The life of most married women centres round the looking after of their husband, children and home. To many it is the purpose and end of their life, the object of all their hopes and ambitions, the vehicle for their energies and enthusiasm. Suddenly to ask these women to give up their children is like asking a keen physician to give up his practice or a naval captain his ship. They will feel bored and miserable.

As a result of evacuating the children many a house-wife left in the danger areas has felt both lonely and bored. It is true that few of them would like their children to be in London if bombs were dropped. But this does not mean to say that the majority are happy remaining on without them. We must not forget that a large number of people find being left alone in a house a very great strain. They feel desperately lonely and frightened. This may be irrational but we can neither ignore it, nor blame those who suffer from it. The presence of a child may make all the difference between cheerful activity and anxious depressed moping. And fathers must not be forgotten. One man of forty went completely off his food when his little girl was sent away. He ate nothing and got more and more depressed. After two or three weeks of this it was hardly surprising that his wife brought the child back again.

Many parents are prepared to admit that these were the reasons why they brought their children home. Others rationalise and invent reasons that will be less condemned – that the child was unhappy or in bad billets. But even if these were often excuses we must admit that some of the children have been very unhappy and have been in bad billets. It is true that parents' fears are often unjustified. But what parent has not some unjustified fears?

Another common reason for parents taking their children home again has been a fear of their alienation. In the cases of infants and toddlers, this fear is fully justified as has been explained in the previous section. In the case of older children it may be less justified but even so it may be impossible for an anxious mother not to feel worried lest her treasures should come to prefer their foster-homes and foster-mothers. Very many children have been taken away from foster-homes because the standard of living was too good and the parents have been afraid of their children making comparisons unfavourable to themselves. Such action may not be admirable but it is very natural and understandable.

The point I wish to make here is that human nature is irrational and contrary. One mother I came across complained alternately that her children were being badly looked after and so would suffer and that they were being so well looked after that they would not want to return to her. Such worries may be absurd and they may be ungrounded but it is only human for people to have these anxieties and no good comes from ignoring and jeering at them.

An altogether different aspect of the problem relating to the parents whose children have been evacuated is that of the mother who does not want her children back. The headmaster of an elementary school taking children from very poor parts reports that many of the children's mothers have taken the opportunity to get work and supplement the family income. Others have always resented the responsibility of children and are glad to be rid of them. When the time comes for the children to be compulsorily returned emotional and economic problems arising from this quarter must be expected.

Foster-parents also have many psychological problems but in this very short survey there is no space to consider them.

Recommendations

Having now briefly surveyed some of the emotional problems which either have or are likely to arise as a result of evacuation we can make some practical proposals. In the first place the mere recognition of a problem may take us half way to solving it. If we realise that a child is feeling anxious about his parents some discussion of what is really happening in the cities may be a great help to him. If we recognise that much bedwetting, disobedience, temper tantrums and other habits are due to anxiety and homesickness, we shall avoid punitive measures and do what we can to reassure the child. Again if we can see things from the point of view of the foster-mother or the bereaved parent instead of condemning and bullying them, we are likely to help them more to adapt to the peculiarly difficult circumstances in which they find themselves.

In the second place it is necessary to sound a note of warning about camps. Unless large numbers of experienced workers can be found to run them they will not provide the homely background which the younger children undoubtedly require. Moreover, as the Cambridge Survey has shown, the majority of the children placed in foster-homes are tolerably well off. The analysis of school reports and friendly visitor's reports on how the children were getting on in their billets showed that about three-quarters of them were reasonable happy and contented. In only twenty five of the 300 cases were the relations of foster-mother and child seriously bad.

For those children who are admittedly intolerable in foster-homes small homes should be set up. Groups of up to twenty children can be catered for and the house run on homely lines. They should be under the supervision of someone experienced in the management of difficult children and staffed by kindly sensible people who are prepared for the difficulties which looking after such children entails.

Much of the ordinary billeting can continue to be done by amateur workers. Nevertheless it should be realised that the successful placement of children in foster-homes requires skill, training and experience. Some of the voluntary workers who have undertaken it have this experience but many have none. For this reason it is a very serious criticism of the Government's Evacuation Scheme that no attempt has ever been made to enlist the services of social workers whose peace-time profession it is to handle problems of this kind. The Committee of the Cambridge Evacuation Survey[1] have strongly recommended the appointment of trained professional social workers, many of whom are at present idle, to help in the organisation of billeting. They recommend that one full-time and responsible person be available for every 500 children.

The management of difficult and nervous children requires even more skill and experience. In certain areas social workers with special training in mental health have been engaged and it is to be hoped that more will be

1 [Bowlby notes:] Memorandum on Practical Recommendations, March 21st, 1940, available from Hon. Sec. Evacuation Research Committee, 30, Causewayside, Cambridge.

utilised. The Ministry of Health is sympathetic to these appointments and will consider reimbursing Local Authorities who engage them.[2]

Finally we must consider arrangements for small children under five years of age – one of the most difficult and debatable of issues.[3] The very great dangers to small children of being moved away from their mothers to the care of strangers for long periods has already been stressed. Let us then first arrange that suitable accommodation is available in the country for those mothers who wish to go with their children. There will be many mothers whose husbands are in the forces who would be evacuated with their babies if bombing became serious, provided proper accommodation were available. Billeting them in other people's houses has proved a complete failure, but wherever empty houses have been made available, satisfactory arrangements have been made. Empty cottages are of course very scarce, but there are two other possibilities. In the first place it might be possible to take over large houses in safe areas and adapt them so that they could be used to accommodate a community of small families. The mothers would do the work and look after the children. Secondly the construction of special encampments might be considered – a policy which the Society of Friends is advocating.

Where mothers cannot be evacuated with their toddlers, the children should only be sent away when it is absolutely necessary. In these cases any nurses and helpers specially recruited should be appointed as *foster-mothers to particular children* instead of nurses to an institution. By appointing them as foster-mothers a definite relationship is implied and the worker is encouraged to remain responsible for a given child's welfare. In these circumstances permanent emotional relations can be hoped for between the child and the worker. Even so no child under two should be evacuated without his mother unless to close personal friends. This view has now been accepted in official quarters, for, apart from the psychological dangers involved, there are great problems of the physical care and management of large numbers of babies.

Conclusion

In conclusion then let us recognise that by evacuating children and others from the danger areas we are having great emotional as well as economical problems and that these problems cannot be met simply by blaming people

2 [Bowlby notes:] Names of suitable workers can be obtained from the Mental Health Emergency Committee, 24, Buckingham Palace Road, S.W.1.
3 [Bowlby notes:] This and other psychological problems are dealt with more fully in "Children in War-Time", March 1940, obtainable from the New Era, 29, Tavistock Square, W.C.1., price 7d.

for being unreasonable. We have first to take the trouble to understand and to make allowances for human nature. We must recognise that there are some children who are quite unsuitable to leave their parents, there are others who are quite unsuitable to be put in someone else's home; there are foster-parents who should not have the care of children and there are parents whose children ought not to be taken from them.

Experience however suggests that these cases are the exception and that with skilled work and the wise choice of foster-mothers the majority of children can be settled fairly satisfactorily in foster-homes. It is a mistake to think that because there have been so many failures there are no successes. Putting children under 12 in camps is not a good solution and everything should be done to make the foster-home placement a success. Workers skilled in this exist and their services should be widely utilised, especially as the Ministry of Health are prepared to pay for them.

There is no evidence that children over five are likely to suffer serious psychological harm from being sent away, although already unstable children may get worse and the normal children may be unhappy and homesick.

There are grave reasons, however, for fearing that sending children under 5 away from their homes, to be looked after for long months at a time by complete strangers, may cause serious emotional disturbances. For this reason it is advocated that no children under 5 be evacuated without their mothers unless serious raids make it essential. Even then no child under 2 years should go. When children between 2 and 5 years of age are evacuated without their mothers the very greatest of care should be taken to see that whoever looks after them remains with them. Without this precaution there is a danger that the child will develop into a seriously anti-social and criminal character.

Bed-wetting

Bedwetting is probably the commonest disorder of behaviour met with among the evacuated children and it is almost certainly the most trying to the foster mother. In some areas it has been estimated that as many as 60% of the children have developed this distressing symptom.

In attempting to deal with the problem *a careful distinction must be made between the child who has developed the habit since evacuation and the child who has had it for years.* The latter, who is usually well-known to his schoolmasters, calls for special care and treatment which usually takes a long time and may be met with much discouragement, though eventually success is nearly always obtained.

The majority, however, have wet their beds only since coming away from home and it is safe to say that the disorder is rarely the result of lack of training as many are tempted to think. It is not just laziness either, nor "naughtiness" except on a few isolated occasions, nor is the root cause likely to be a "weak" bladder or kidneys or too much to drink at night. In these cases the cause nearly always lies either in the child's physical environment or in his feelings of shyness and homesickness.

Certain obvious factors present themselves: the lavatory may be dark and terrifying to a nervous child in a strange house and he may fail to go there before retiring, or he may be afraid to get out of bed during the night. An imaginative child, feeling insecure in strange surroundings, will people the darkness around him with the most terrifying inhabitants even without being told stories by unwise adults. He may be shy of his foster mother and so fail to prepare himself for bed properly. Again he may be cold in bed or dislike getting out into the cold to relieve himself.

But there are many children in whom no single reason of this sort is found. The child, in spite of his best endeavours, wets himself. One way of regarding it is to think of it as a return to babyhood. Those who themselves have brought up young children will recall how after dry habits have been established relapses will occur at such times as the arrival of another baby, a strange child in the house, a move or change in the adults about him, or on first going to school. The interpretation may be that by returning to babyhood he may again set first claim on the attentions of his mother. This rarely, if ever, a conscious thought and most children would be exceedingly ashamed of such ideas and would never admit having them, even to themselves. Again bed-wetting is sometimes an expression of sadness and it must be remembered that many evacuated children are far more homesick than they let others know.

It must be remembered that while the foster mother has all the vexation of extra washing and ruining of the mattresses and the worry lest there be something seriously wrong, a sensitive child will suffer agonies of shame from this relapse to dirtiness and from the consciousness or fear of adult disapproval. This will naturally increase the conflict already present in the child's mind.

Bearing in mind this explanation of the commonest causes of bed-wetting, the general principles of dealing with individual children are quite straightforward.

1) Of fundamental importance is the selection of an understanding and calm foster mother who is capable of feeling real love for her charges; and it is vital for lasting success to provide just that love and security that the child has been lacking since being torn so suddenly from his own family. Such a foster mother will see the unwisdom of a disciplinary attitude as only increasing the child's difficulties, will be encouraging, and will show by her manner that she expects the child to get better sooner or later and does not reject him from her affections because of his dirtiness. The foster mother herself will need

support and encouragement in this attitude, because hers is a very difficult and trying task. The foster-mother who approaches the task in a spirit of missionary zeal is unlikely to be successful. She easily becomes disappointed and dispirited and vents her feelings on the children.

2) Hot tea or milk is to be avoided during the hour before going to bed. Systematic abstention from any liquid during the afternoon is quite unnecessary and rather cruel.

3) Care should be taken to see that the child is really warm and comfortable in bed. The provision of extra blankets and a hot water bottle may save much trouble.

4) Simple measures should be taken to make it easy for the child to use the lavatory or the chamber both before and, if necessary, during the night. If the child is expected to go to the lavatory, a night light should be left on or care taken to show him where the light switches are. If a chamber is provided a little bit of matting on which to kneel or stand makes the operation more comfortable.

In certain areas where these measures have been taken over three-quarters of the cases of bed-wetting have cleared up.

Two courses in particular are to be avoided.

1) Continual changes in foster-homes each time reproduce afresh many of the conditions making for bed-wetting. Shyness, ignorance of the position of light switches and above all the uncertainty created by being pushed from pillar to post are inevitable during the first few days at each billet.

2) Segregation of bed-wetters in large special homes makes some children worse. The child who is not a chronic case, but who has taken to wetting the bed as a result of the upheaval of evacuation, will find none of the security and reassurance which he needs in a large home. He will become more miserable and the bed-wetting will continue.

Chronic cases

Those children who had wet their beds regularly even before the evacuation are in a minority. Sympathetic enquiries from brothers and sisters or school teachers will usually establish their identity. For these cases there is no simple remedy. They should only be taken on by foster-mothers who understand quite clearly that they will have to put up with the symptom and that they are unlikely to get the satisfaction of seeing an improvement. Only a special type of woman should be asked to undertake such a task. Many such children would be better off at home even in a danger area than in safety but with unsuitable foster-mothers.

The uprooted small child

When the effects upon children of a domestic upheaval or a family tragedy are being discussed, one often hears the remarks: "Oh he's only a little chap – fortunately it won't affect him" or "Of course he was too young to understand". In these statements it is implied that the very small child is far less influenced by family events than his older brothers and sisters, who may be expected to be upset and troubled. This view has often been challenged and nowadays is challenged by the great majority of child psychologists. Small children have a most deceptive way of appearing not to be affected by these events. A beloved nurse may leave and the child never even refers to her again. Mother goes abroad and the child appears to settle cheerfully and happily with someone else. Surely evidence of this kind proves that small children are not affected. Why should anyone think otherwise?

In the first place it must be remembered that all small children, by which I mean children between twelve months and five years, do not settle down happily after their mothers or nurses have left them. Sometimes in fact they mope so much and eat so little that mother or nurse has to be sent for. At other times they become troublesome and difficult and no one can quite understand why the sweet-tempered has become so irritable and tiresome. And besides the children who show these unmistakeable signs of unhappiness and distress, careful observation of many of those who appear not to be affected shows that underneath their cheerful exterior they are minding very much indeed. Sometimes the child who never mentions the nurse who has left him will play a game in which the nurse appears as a cruel and horrid person who deserted her baby. The child whose mother has gone abroad will play games about little children whose mother has died. Often to a sympathetic person a great deal of unhappiness and anxiety is expressed in this kind of way. The fact that a child settles down with strangers often means no more than that he has become resigned to his fate. He believes himself an orphan, for ever deserted by those he has loved and trusted. Efforts to find them and get back to them are therefore useless. He gives up hope and makes the best of a bad job. This despairing frame of mind may persist through life. Viewed in this way we can see that it is really a misfortune that small children become resigned so easily, for if they protested more violently many injurious things would not be done. For we are now beginning to learn that many harmful things can be done to a baby and a toddler without its being obvious at the time, just as the effects of bad diet may take months or even years to manifest itself.

Those who work in child guidance clinics and see many heinous, difficult and delinquent children are all too often faced with the after-results of these long separations. A remarkably high proportion of such children are found to have had most unsettled home conditions during their first few years of life. Sometimes their mother was ill or died and they were looked after by a succession of different people. Sometimes their parents were abroad and they were left in the hands of strange aunts and nurses, sometimes the parents separated, sometimes the child himself was in hospital. But, whatever the cause, the striking thing about these children's lives has been that in their early years they have been for periods of many months in the hands of complete strangers instead of in the unchanged care of one or two familiar women as most children are.

And if we investigate these cases further we often find that as a result of these changes and long separations the child has become completely estranged from his mother. For instance one little boy who had been in hospital unvisited from the age of 15 months until he was 2 years old had completely failed to recognise his mother on his return home.

He insisted on calling her "nurse" and refused anything to eat for several days. Apart from the effect on the child such a state of affairs is naturally very distressing for the mother. No doubt many children who have suffered these experiences regain contact with their families afterward, but there can be no doubt that many do not. When this happens the child is apt to grow up into a discontented and difficult adolescent and to be a chronic social misfit in later life. For if a child is not happy and on good terms with his own family he commonly fails to be happy and on good terms with anyone else. As a warning it may be remarked that Goering apparently suffered an experience of this kind when he was three. It is by no means fanciful to supposed that this event was responsible for his growing into the violent and ruthless character which we now know.

Reflections of this kind are obviously most relevant at the present day when we are planning for the evacuation of large numbers of small children. If we face the dangers squarely there is no reason why they should not be overcome but if we try to pretend that there is no problem and think that so long as he is "too young to understand" it does not much matter what we arrange we shall certainly make mistakes of a far-reaching kind.

What then are we to do about it? What practical steps can we take which will avoid, or at least reduce, the risks described?

In the first place every encouragement should be given to mothers to leave the danger areas with their small children so that they can continue looking after them themselves. There can be no doubt that this is the ideal course from the child's point of view, although as we all now know there are many practical difficulties to be overcome. Even if they will leave their homes, mothers with babies present a great problem to the Billeting officers. With the best will in the world few women can share their house with another. There is friction over small things and they get on each other's nerves. In almost every case where a mother and baby has been billeted in someone else's house they have gone home. The few mothers who have remained are almost all housed in empty cottages and wings of houses. In these they appear to be very happy, and if more accommodation of this kind could be provided it seems reasonable to suppose that a large number of mothers with small children would be willing to be evacuated again.

But unfortunately empty cottages and houses are scarce. An experiment might reasonably be tried however of taking over large empty houses where available and arranging them so they could be occupied by a community of evacuated mothers and children. A warden would probably be necessary but all the work of the house and care of the children would be left in the hands of the mothers. The Government might also be urged to build cottage camps for mothers and children instead of school camps, but this proposal lies outside the scope of this article.

First then let us do our best to arrange accommodation for however many mothers care to accompany their children. It is of course more difficult and far more nuisance to provide accommodation for mothers as well as for children but there can be no doubt that it is in the children's interest to do so.

But there are of course many, probably a majority, of mothers who for one reason or another cannot accompany their young children. Many have husbands and homes to look after, some have older adolescent children to provide for. They feel that they cannot leave. Yet they want their two, three and four-year olds out of the danger area.

One solution of this problem has been found by parents finding friends or relations for their children to go with or stay with, for it is far less of a shock for a small child to be looked after by someone he knows than by a complete and total stranger. If an aunt, a granny or an old family friend already living in a safe area will take the child so much the better. When this is not possible mothers should be encouraged to find a friend or neighbour who is being evacuated and would look after an extra baby. This was done to some extent last September. In some cases unmarried girls who were friends of the family under-took to look after the toddlers. This plan might be explored further since by utilising the mothers who are prepared to leave the cities to look after their friends' three years olds as well as their own, some at least of the emotional problems could be avoided. This scheme however depends upon adequate and suitable accommodation being provided in the billeting areas.

Finally we come to the crucial problem. What is to be done with the thousands of toddlers whose mothers can neither take them themselves nor find friends or relations who can take them?

First let it be said that it is far better that the real babies should not go at all. Any baby under two years is quite unfit to be sent away from his mother unless it be to close and reliable friends. This view seems now to be held in official circles and there can be no doubt it is the right one.

Moreover so long as there are no air-raids there are powerful reasons for leaving the two, three and four year olds in the danger areas with their mothers. Unlike the older children who at the most are coming to no serious harm and who at the best are profiting greatly from their experiences, very young children away from their mothers with strangers for months at a time may suffer severe psychological damage. To run this risk, when there is no bombing seems foolish. It would be tragic if more damage were to be caused by our precautions than by the weapons they were designed to protect us against.

Nevertheless many people will not share this view. Moreover air-raids may begin at any moment and we must have a clear policy. Plans for the evacuation of children in large groups and day nurseries have mercifully been abandoned although a number of children are still being cared for in this way. Instead, the placing of children in foster homes is being considered. Where willing foster mothers can be found there can be not doubt that this is the best policy although it may be difficult to accommodate sufficient numbers in this way.

If all else fails it may be necessary to evacuate some of them in the care of trained workers. But whether it be a country woman or a trained worker who looks after the children certain vital precautions are necessary if the worst results are to be avoided.

Very serious attention should be given to *see that the children remain in the care of one woman, who should always bear the official title of foster-mother.* By so describing her the proper emotional relation is encouraged and she is encouraged too to regard the children to some extent her own. She is far more likely to feel responsible for the child's future and so to remain with her particular charges for the duration of the war.

It must be repeated that it is very bad for small children to be looked after by a succession of strange people. If small children must be evacuated to the care of strangers in the midst of strange surroundings, all that is humanly possible should be done to see that the stranger who takes them remains with them. It must be remembered that the changes from mother to foster-mother and back again from foster-mother to mother at the end of the war constitute two great emotional upheavals in the little child's development. These two changes are bad enough though they may be unavoidable. But when a child is in a resident nursery and looked after first by one person and then by another, no one person looking after him all the time, then the likelihood of damage is infinitely increased. The same of course is true if a child changes frequently from one foster-home to another.

What can and should be avoided therefore is placing little children in large groups under the care of a matron and endlessly changing junior nurses. A staff of this kind may be very admirable in its work and genuinely kind to the children. But not having a special relation to a few individual children the nurses are not in a position to provide that solid personal background which small children so much need if they are to grow up into happy and sociable human beings. For the same reasons changes from one foster-mother to another are at all costs to be avoided.

If on the contrary the organisation is planned so that the women helpers are appointed not as nurses to an institution but as foster-mothers to particular children the dangers we are concerned with would be largely avoided. The foster-mother would be with her little family during the day as their ordinary mother would. She would get them up and dress them, give them their meals, play with them, bath them. It is in these everyday activities that emotional bonds are forged between a grown up and a child. Naturally the foster-mother would want the help of a nursemaid like any other mother with several young children. The nursemaid could be quite inexperienced and untrained but would be capable of doing much of the heavier work and, with guidance, of looking after the children when the foster-mother had time off. Moreover the new Nursery Centres which are being set up in various areas should give the foster-mother, whether married women in the country or specially appointed workers some rest from their labours during the day.

Finally the question of the mother's visits is an important one. In some hospitals mothers are not encouraged to visit their small children because of the tears shed on their departure. It is certainly inconvenient for the nurses and distressing for the children, but this does not necessarily mean that it is bad for them. Indeed experience suggests that is is the children who are not visited and who consequently completely forget their parents who in the long run fare the worst. The younger the child the more frequent the visits should be and even for children of three, visits should not be less frequent than monthly. These regular visits will not only smooth the way for the return home after hostilities have ceased but will go far to maintain the normal emotional contact between mother and child which it is believed is of such outstanding importance for the welfare of the little child.

To sum up therefore we should recommend:

(1) that suitable accommodation should be provided in reception areas for those mothers who are willing to go with their younger children. Such accommodation should not be in other people's houses, but should provide the evacuated mother with a little home of her own either in an empty house or as part of a community of mothers and children in a large house. Village camps should also be pressed for.

(2) In the case of children whose mothers cannot leave the danger areas, every effort should be made to arrange for them to go either to friends or relations already in a safe area or with friends who are themselves being evacuated.

(3) Where this cannot be arranged it should be considered whether the child is not better off with his mother in a danger area than in a safe area with a stranger. Babies under two years old should on no account be evacuated to the care of strangers.

(4) If small children are evacuated without either mothers or friends, every possible care should be taken to see that they remain in the care of one person during the period of their evacuation. To this end it is suggested that as many children as possible should be placed in families with willing foster-mothers, but that where special workers are employed these workers should be appointed as foster-mothers to particular children instead of as nurses to a large group of children. In this way it is hoped to encourage a sense of personal interest and responsibility to individual children amongst the helpers.

(5) Every encouragement should be given to mothers to visit their little children regularly, if possible at least monthly.

Chapter 6

Freud and the super-ego

[Editors' note: undated handwritten text, likely from 1933–1936. Wellcome Library Archive PP/BOW/D.2/49]

The ego is complicated. Its nucleus is perception-consciousness, with the special senses connected with its own body – the kinaesthetic senses – as its ultimate kernel. Its function is to test reality and in so doing it stores within itself memories of the external world in all its aspects. Thus one may say that a person's ego is constructed from their sensory experience of the external world. This everyday phenomenon appears to me to have essentially the same characteristics as the process of introjection which Freud, I believe, limits to the process of incorporating the libido's object.

Naturally the libido's object is especially important and when it is built into the ego it has a far greater influence than other objects. The process of building in objects and impressions leads to the ego reacting to new situations in certain characteristic ways. But some of these objects are incompatible with others which produces a conflict of reactions and the tendency of some to go to the wall.

A particularly incompatible and indigestible incorporation are the parents. The feelings associated with the Oedipus complex are very strong and always conflicting; for a certain amount of satisfaction is gained from them and so they are loved, but in so far as they do not provide satisfaction either implicitly or explicitly they are hated. The set of reactions developing from this forms the nucleus of the super-ego. It is a protective mechanism in the ego designed to avoid the criticisms of the parents. It does this by tabooing all feelings and desires which cannot be fulfilled and which if attempted would lead to punishment. It is therefore naturally modelled on the restrictions and permissions of the parents and partakes of their characters. This is another way of saying that the parents are introjected.

Now this super-ego behaves in a peculiarly ruthless way and derives from consciousness feelings and desires which are incompatible with it. They not only become unconscious by the mechanism of repression but the super-ego is constantly concerned to resist their entry into consciousness. Since the super-ego, and the ego of which it is a part, control motility these desires are not expressed in action, unless the ego itself is so split by the incompatibility of its elements that the desire is able to find some sympathetic part of the ego to translate it into action.

It is this split in the ego which is all-important in the development of character. If the super-ego is so incompatible with other parts of the ego which are used to giving gratification then the super-ego is itself repressed from consciousness, but none the less continues its functions most of the time. It is then felt as an external force and therefore projected.

It appears that the repression of libidinal desires occurs when the super-ego dominates consciousness in childhood and that it itself is only repressed later when its prohibitions are felt as intolerable by new structures dominating consciousness. If this is so, repression is a function of consciousness whilst resistance may proceed from unconscious material. A faulty development of the libido occurs when the inhibitions imposed by the super-ego so hamper object-choice that gratification is impossible. When this happens the libido either attempts gratification by some circuitous route or else is driven to obtain it through earlier channels.

It is largely in terms of this repression and fixation of libido interest that psychoanalysis explains personality, finding the causes of such fixations in faulty ego development.

Super-ego

Functions

(1) To provide the ego with a series of data as to how other people may be expected to behave in relation to the self.
(2) To instruct the ego how to behave towards these people in order to preserve the self from danger.

    (a) by protesting to the ego against certain forms of behaviour promoted by the id, and threatening the ego with punishment in order to prevent it carrying out such actions. (Is the super-ego responsible for carrying out this punishment upon the self, or does the ego do this?)
    (b) by exhorting the ego towards certain other actions and ideals.

To say that the super-ego consists of the identifications of the parents means:

(1) That the data in question is founded chiefly upon what the parents were believed to be like.

    (a) That the behaviour proscribed will be similar to that of the "bad" parents and that the protests and threats will resemble those "used" by the parents.

(b) That the behaviour demanded will approximate to the behaviour of the 'good' parents.

In the "Ego & Id", Freud describes what he believes to be the origin of the *super-ego* (Freud, 1923b, p.44) as a special modification of the ego – consisting of the Oedipus identifications of the ego in some way fused together, and he describes its function (Freud, 1923b, p.45) as having "the task of effecting the repression of the Oedipus complex."

This may be true but its origin seems to be earlier than Freud first supposed for Mrs Klein finds unmistakeable signs of its activities, such as guilt and self-punishment, in children in their second year.

In consequence although the task of repressing the Oedipus complex may be an important function of the super-ego, it is no longer possible to consider it either as its original or only purpose.

Mrs Klein has in consequence put forward an other alternative hypothesis first suggested by Freud in "Instincts and their Vicissitudes" (Freud, 1915c) namely that it is formed as a controller of the child's sadism.

It seems to me profitable to take this as our starting point.

Now the function of the ego is to form a series of paths by which id impulses can be discharged in accordance with the reality principle. An important part of this function is the temporary delaying of discharge until circumstances are suitable. This system is built up according to certain patterns which are recommended to the child either explicitly or implicitly by its parents. So as soon as such a system is working smoothly it probably becomes temporarily unconscious and the activities of consciousness are taken up with reactions whose appropriateness is more open to doubt.

Now one of the first impulses which has to be delayed by the ego is aggression, which it seems to me is most simply regarded as the natural reaction of the organism to frustration. Whether this delay is due to the disapproval with which parents regard all signs of aggression or to internal causes I am at present uncertain.

However, the child at a very early age becomes afraid of its own aggression towards its love-objects and learns to avoid its expression. Now this is in itself a perfectly typical action of the *ego*, in the same way that an adult ego will forgo a lesser gratification for a greater. The question now becomes, why does this particular reaction of the ego, which seems to be originally so typical of ordinary ego functions, become so disjointed from the ordinary ego, and go through such a curious development of its own?

Normally, delayed impulses are held waiting consciously in the ego, awaiting an opportunity of expression. The impulse to urinate and defecate is delayed for instance until a time when it will be regarded by the parents as right and proper. Even sexual desires, so long delayed, are appreciated by the child as being possible for adults to gratify.

Aggression however differs from all these.

In the first place it is regarded by many parents as being universally bad. Second, the child apprehends that its instincts to destroy its object will prevent its other desires being gratified. It is perhaps because of the apparent impossibility of gratifying this impulse that, like all other certainties, it gets relegated to unconsciousness and fails to modify its expression as most other id impulses do via the ego. This is a possible explanation for the initial splitting of the super-ego reactions from the ego. How does it develop?

A striking feature of the super-ego is the way in which the child identifies it with his parents. The origin of this seems to be in the three mechanisms

(1) The super-ego is *partly* formed at the parent's behest and in obedience to them. Not surprisingly perhaps the child mistakes one factor for the sum of factors.

(2) This mistake would be supported by the child's early difficulty in distinguishing itself from others. By means of this wrong identification (introjection) it regards prohibitions which it has itself imposed as coming from without, especially since so many prohibitions do come from without.

(3) Since it has in fact had the desire to incorporate its parents, really it is not surprising that it should imagine that the inhibition, which it feels, springs immediately from an oral incorporation actually performed.

In these various ways then the super-ego becomes on the one hand the unconscious prototype of all further instinct inhibitions and also is endowed with all the properties attributable to parents. If this view is correct the super-ego can be regarded as an alter-ego which is remarkable in the first place for its drastic repression of a certain portion of the id and secondly from the fact that since it itself remains unconscious it fails to develop and retains the stamp of parental authority.

Thus its relation to the id is similar to the ego's relation to it. Furthermore, it seems to me possible that its identity to parents may well be shared with the infantile ego. Thus it seems not unlikely that the whole infantile ego organisation has a parental quality derived, as much of it is, from parental example and precept and that normally this specifically parental quality is gradually transmuted in the real ego whereas the super-ego remaining unconscious retains this quality much later in life.

To recapitulate:

(1) Impulses of aggression towards the love object are inhibited in the usual ego-way.

(2) This early organisation becomes especially identified with the parents.

Ego, super-ego and ego-ideal

These terms must be considered from the point of view of *FUNCTION*.

ID. = (animal needs) biological needs, shared with lower creatures.
These needs vary during the individual's lifetime *and* according to the environment.

> *Maturation* of biological needs e.g., changes in sex behaviour
> changes in food appetites
> changes in behaviour
> vis à vis enemies
> (submission, aggression)

> *Environmental influence* e.g., in sex – presence of wife and children
> in self-protection– nature of enemies

sex
food   } lead in childhood to ally with parents
self-protection   }   "   "
protection of children   }   "   "

SUPER-EGO. = maintenance of social relations
– fundamental function designed to maintain satisfactory relations with parents – a necessity due to the infant's helplessness. In our socialised society later becomes the function maintaining good relations with the social group or God.

> *Maturation*
> nature of super-ego will vary with child's age and the degree of his dependence on parents and later on society.

> *Environmental influence – real and fancied*
> (a) parent's demands (Cs and Ucs)[1]
> (b) traumas such as separation, sudden deaths, etc.
> (c) demands of social group, e.g., different class demands
> (d) demands of particular loved individuals e.g., schoolmasters.

---

1 [Editors' note:] Cs is shorthand for conscious. Ucs is shorthand for unconscious.

It is useful to consider the super-ego as essentially that part of the ego which is concerned to maintain social relations. It will be motivated by a desire for the benefits which the object provides (food, protection, sex, etc.), which complements the fear of losing these benefits (fear of loss of love) and *secondarily* by altruistic love which is closely bound up with identification with the object.

Egalitarianism, justice, honesty, democracy etc. can all be regarded as techniques for maintaining good social relations – and minimising intra-group tensions. They can therefore be inferred from the proposition that to live efficiently organisms require to have friendly relations with others.

Each society values certain virtues – all have in common the valuation of some degree of loyalty. Those virtues which are valued are those which are *believed* by the people to make for social cohesion. Sometimes this is really the case, in others not so. Once a virtue comes to be valued, whether with good reason or not, it comes to have a certain independent social status and becomes a *cultural ideal* and may also acquire an independent status for the individual.

EGO-IDEAL = organism's long-term aims

> Long term aims normally selected by the organism as being consistent with its capabilities and inclination and also with the super-ego demands. (NB., If those demands are very severe or incompatible with the organism's capabilities, a satisfactory ego-ideal will not be formed).

> *Maturation*
>> with changes in (a) animal needs, (b) abilities and (c) in social demands, nature of long-term aims will change.

> *Environmental influence*
>> (a) influenced by cultural ideals of group
>> (b) by individual members, e.g., parents and schoolmasters, who advise on desirable levels of aspiration
>> (c) opportunities

> *Internal influences*   evaluational facilities
>> (a) ego-phantasies – beliefs (Cs or Ucs, realistic or unrealistic) regarding own nature and abilities
>> (b) nature of super-ego

The operation of environmental influences will depend on the organism's selective action. An intelligent child may respond to proposals which will leave another child cold.

Both the super-ego and the ego-ideal are functions which *control* the immediate short term impulses of the individual. One controls them in the interests of preserving good social relations, the other in the interest of achieving personal long-term aims.

Ego

The function which controls motor activity. It decides which dynamic system is to have access to the motor activity (including thought processes) at any given time. The burden of decision is greatly alleviated by *routine*.

Cs, "free-will", etc. belong to the ego. Much of the selective and controlling functions of the ego occur unconsciously.

References

Freud, S. (1915c). *Instincts and their Vicissitudes. S. E., 14*: 111–140. London: Hogarth Press.

Freud, S. (1923b). *The Ego and the Id. S. E., 19*: 3–66. London: Hogarth Press.

Chapter 7

Guilt and family contracts

[Editors: Handwritten manuscript, undated but likely c.1937–1939. Title added by the editors. Wellcome Collection Archive PP/BOW/D.1/2/13]

In *Civilisation and its Discontents*, Freud (1930a, pp.105–109) deals with the problem of guilt in some detail. He begins with the premise that people feel guilty when they have done something which they know to be bad. He then asks how is it that we know what is bad and concludes that, since evil is not always that which would endanger the ego, there must be some extraneous influence. This influence he believes to be the dread of losing love. From this he argues back to the nature of evil and says "What is bad is, therefore, to begin with, whatever causes one to be threatened with a loss of love." He points out that this may be either a wish or a deed. But at this stage he thinks it improper to call it a sense of guilt. It is "only the dread of losing love, 'social' anxiety". But he maintains "a great change takes place as soon as the authority has been internalised by the development of a super-ego." "At this point the dread of discovery ceases to operate" and the terms conscience and guilt are truly applicable.

Before following Freud's arguments further I want to examine these conclusions, upon which so much else rests. In the first place, as Freud himself agrees, it is incorrect to say that we feel guilty because we have done something which might lead to loss of love. On the contrary there are occasions when we feel it to be right to do something which will lead to disapproval. And if this is so, his statement that what is bad is whatever causes one to be threatened with a loss of love is manifestly incorrect. It is true in some instances and not in others and consequently will not do as a definition of what is bad. There is however an important element of truth in Freud's statement, which will be examined again later. For the present I cannot accept it as a definition or even approximate definition of what is bad. Consequently his description of the internalisation of the sense of guilt is unsatisfactory and needs to be re-examined.

Later in the book, however, Freud puts forward a different theory which he arrives at after a consideration of his phylogenetic theories. He argues that a sense of guilt first arose when the sons had killed the primal father and then regretted it. This leads to the conclusion that guilt is the expression of the conflict of ambivalence, the fear of destroying that which one loves. He points out that no punishment is to be expected after the primal father's death and that the sense of guilt is purely internal, dependent upon self-condemnation, not external condemnation.

Before discussing the validity of the general theory that guilt is the result of ambivalence, it is as well to point out that after the death of someone to whom a patient has felt ambivalent we regularly find the very real expectation of their ghost returning to haunt them. Yet there can be no doubt however that people do feel guilty even when no sort of retribution is to be expected and this will need examination.

Is guilt always the expression of a conflict of ambivalence? I don't think that it is. In the first place there are occasions when guilt is experienced when no ambivalence is present – neither love nor hate. Supposing that I met a stranger in the country and the stranger asked me to post a letter for him. I promise to do so, thinking that it will be little bother to me and a service to him. Such a feeling hardly deserves the name love; indeed he might be a little repulsive to me. A week later I find the letter still in my pocket. This would make me feel guilty because I had broken my promise, not because I had inconvenienced someone whom I love.

Furthermore I suspect that there are consciously ambivalent interactions where no guilt is experienced. There are many people whom one likes in part and dislikes in part, varying perhaps from day to day. Provided that one is honest about it and do not mislead them I don't think that guilt is felt.

Consequently I cannot accept Freud's theory of guilt – that it "is the expression of the conflict of ambivalence," (Freud, 1930a, p. 121) though it cannot be questioned that guilt is extremely frequently felt in an ambivalent relationship. What seems to be the case is that guilt is felt when there is a *pretence* that the hatred does not exist and there is an implicit *promise* of love. This, of course, is the common condition when the ambivalence is unconscious. To my mind therefore it is not the ambivalence itself which constitutes the grounds for guilt, but guilt is experienced only when we *fail to do what we have undertaken to do*. Unconscious ambivalence is a special instance of the more general theory; if we have undertaken to love a person, we naturally feel guilty if we find ourselves hating them. This theory that we feel guilty when we break our undertaking, some kind of contract, seems to me to account for a great many facts.

We know that it is impossible to discover any particular deed which all men would agree was always bad. Murder and robbery are usually condemned, but during wartime they are considered good. Why are they considered good during war and not in peace? In 1914 this country was roused to righteous anger because Germany broke a treaty which she had solemnly signed. The sanctity of treaties was regarded as of far more moral importance than millions of human lives and no deed was considered too bad to punish this crime, provided again we had made no promise to refrain from using it. For instance, we had promised not to use poison gas and we thought it would be *wrong* to use poison gas. We only used it when the contract was broken by the enemy. Then it was *right* to use it. Throughout the chaos of moral values of the war years, one principle remained unchanged – *it was wrong to break treaties and contracts.* Whatever else might be right this was universally acknowledged as wrong.

This is inadequate material from which to present a general theory of good and evil. But it seems to me that it is now possible to describe two sets of circumstances in which we feel guilty.

1) When we have broken a promise and fear that this will be discussed and certain results follow.
2) When we have failed to live up to an ideal which we have of ourselves.

The first set of circumstances corresponds to what Freud calls external guilt or social anxiety, the second to what he describes as the internalisation of the authority. Freud recognised that this internalisation depended upon the conditions under which external guilt was experienced and consequently it is desirable to consider the external circumstances first.

"External" guilt

There are occasions when we may fear punishment, but feel such to be unjust. Thus a child considers it unjust if it is beaten for doing something when no one told it not to. It does not feel guilty, but it does feel afraid of the punishment. If the parent maintains that the child has been wicked and that the punishment is just, it is this which provokes the feeling of injustice.

Again there are occasions when severe consequences may ensue but we do not feel guilty. During war time we may regard that it is dangerous to attack the enemy, but we do not feel guilty. External guilt is only warranted when we have failed to keep a promise.

At this point I want to distinguish between rational external guilt and irrational external guilt. People sometimes *feel* guilty when anyone else, knowing the facts, would not think them so. External guilt in my opinion is *only* realistic when a voluntary contract has been broken. Moralised punishment or simple revenge may sometimes follow our actions but no guilt should be called for if no contract has been entered into. This I believe to be the only realistic and objective view of external guilt, although people may feel guilty and *fear* just punishment even when they have not made a promise. If I am right, one problem will then be to discover why people should feel unrealistically guilty.

In considering this question of realistic guilt and unrealistic guilt, I am at present only concerned with external guilt. The problem of realistic and unrealistic internal guilt is an even more difficult problem. The distinction which I am trying to draw is exactly similar to that which we constantly draw between a realistic belief and an unrealistic belief. Thus if a German Jew told us he was persecuted, we should regard it as realistic because there is an overwhelming consensus opinion that it is true. A similar belief on the part of an English Jew, we should regard as very largely unfounded, as unrealistic.

The simplest example of realistic external guilt is when we deliberately break a contract voluntarily entered into. I want a house and sign a lease, promising to pay so much rent for the privilege of living in it. This is a voluntary contract. Supposing now I clear out after getting into arrears with my rent, thereby breaking the contract. Few people would not hold me guilty.

Some headway can now be made in answering Freud's initial questions – how do we know what is bad? I know that it is bad to leave my rent unpaid because I *agreed*, when making the contract, to regard it so. In other words external morality is a matter of social agreement. If two people agree to regard a thing as bad within those limits it is bad. If they agree to regard it as good then it is good.

How then do unrealistic feelings of guilt arise? The commonest and possibly the only way is through contracts being imposed by one party upon another. A noteworthy example of an imposed contract is of course the Versailles Treaty of 1918. The Allies said to Germany "Unless you sign this, we shall hurt you further". Germany consequently signed. In law imposed contracts are invalid, although international law still seems uncertain about it. Even the Catholic church will dissolve a marriage if it is shown that pressure was brought to bear upon one of the parties. It is therefore commonly agreed that no moral stigma or guilt *really* attaches to a person who breaks an imposed contract. But people constantly feel guilty under these conditions, especially children.

When a mother says to a child "I won't love you if you take the jam from the cupboard" and thereby extracts a promise from the child, that is an example of an imposed contract. The child may then steal the jam and will almost certainly feel guilty and fear the threatened punishment, which it regards as *just. Such a feeling of guilt is unrealistic.* In this way I believe very serious warpings of conscience occur.

To sum up our conclusions upon external guilt. The great majority of adults and probably all children feel guilty when they have entered into some kind of contract, either voluntarily or involuntarily, and have broken their part of it.

"Internal" guilt

Internal guilt differs from external guilt inasmuch as no punishment of any kind is to be anticipated. The guilt is wholly internal for we blame *ourselves* for falling short of our *own* ideals. But not any ideal has this result to the same degree. The ideals particularly associated with internal guilt have an interesting property and that is that they have a certain eternal quality. Such an ideal is "to speak the truth *always*". Now how do we come by these ideals and why do we regard them as our own? There seem to me roughly four ways by which they are adopted.

1) In so far as we love and admire our parents we want to be like them and adopt their real or imaginary qualities as our ideals. Thus if my father were to say that it was a good thing to speak the truth I might believe him and do likewise. Such an ideal could be accepted purely voluntarily without threat of any kind. Consequently it could at any time be given up or modified.

2) By voluntary contract. A child may love its parents so much that it voluntarily undertakes to keep an eternal contract. I believe that in practice this voluntary condition occurs far less often than parents pretend.

3) By imposed contract. Under the threat of losing the parents love, a child may make the most ambitious promise, such as a strict temperance pledge. It can be seen that children constantly feel guilty if they break a contract even though it be an imposed one and no guilt is realistically justifiable. Much of the unrealistic guilt experienced by children and adolescents comes from this source, I believe.

4) Our final category of ideals has much in common with category 1, which dealt with ideals directly copied from parents in childhood. But I now wish to deal with those which are consciously and intelligently selected as working rules for living, dictating the behaviour which will in the long run bring us most happiness and satisfaction in life, quite apart from the opinions which other people may hold of us. Thus we may feel that we should like to accomplish a certain task during our life, the achievement of which will produce happiness, but which will entail much hard work. (It will of course always have an unconscious significance as well, but I believe it can also have a realistic significance and it is with that with which I am now dealing). Now if we are lazy and fail to go through with the necessary hard work, we fail to live up to a certain realistic ideal. No punishment is to be expected from outside. The only result of our laziness is that we do not enjoy the fruits which our labours were expected to bring. In other words, we have broken an *implicit contract* with ourselves. Only empirical observation will show, but it is my belief that in so far as our feelings are *realistic* about the task and not implicated by unconscious significance, guilt will not be felt. The feeling would be more akin to disappointment and vexation with ourselves. The reason I think why guilt is not experienced when this contract is broken is because there is no attempt to evade the consequences. Presumably, in this case, were we to deceive ourselves as to the consequences, guilt might be felt.

I do not propose to pursue this speculation further. What emerges however is that ego-ideals can be divided into three big divisions:

Type A) Those voluntarily chosen either in childhood or later life as general rules of that behaviour which will lead to greatest happiness (includes some of group 1 and 2).

Type B) Ideals which have been adopted against our conscious will and in the face of duress and about which we have made no promise (group 2).

Type C) Ideals which form part of a contract entered into either voluntarily or involuntarily, one part of the contract being of an eternal character.

Only the breaking of (C) would lead to guilt.

Contracts

Voluntarily adopted ideals

Although it can be shown that many of our ideals are determined by circumstantial events in our past, it does not follow that all of them are so determined. I do not want to beg the question of free-will or even touch on the many other ethical problems which a discussion of these ideals would necessitate. It is useful to demarcate the boundary between ethics and psycho-analysis however.

Although we may hope for a scientific and unbiased study of ethical ideals in the future, it is clear that at present it is merely a matter of individual judgments and prejudices with much unconscious bias. Therapy grounded upon instilling principles of conduct may or may not be valuable but it is radically different from one which believes that the patient is quite capable of working out his own ethical *Weltanschauung* provided he understands his own wishes and the numerous ideals which either voluntarily or involuntarily he has held on to from his past. We should, I believe, demonstrate under what *contracts* he feels himself to be and so far as we are able to discover whether they were limited or unlimited, voluntary or imposed (see next section). But we are not concerned with the question as to whether unlimited or imposed contracts should, in the present day, be considered binding. If a patient considers that a contract imposed upon him at the age of, say, two is still binding upon him, it is not for us as analysts to disagree, despite the fact that common morality and law would support us: Instead it is because a patient knows it himself, perhaps only vaguely, that it is *unnecessary* to give an opinion about it.

Psycho-analytic therapy specifically avoids dealing with these judgements and voluntarily accepted ideals. They need not therefore be dealt with any further, but left to ethicists and the didactic teachers.

Limited and unlimited contracts

Whether or not these distinctions will help us in understanding case-material has yet to be proved. For the present I intend to continue a theoretical dissection of the conditions under which guilt is felt. So far my argument has led to the conclusion that guilt is experienced when a contract has been made and subsequently broken. Before returning to the distinction between voluntary and imposed contracts, I want to examine further the distinction between limited and unlimited contracts.

What I have hitherto called the sense of external guilt is seen to coincide with the notion of a limited contract. The issue is specific. If I break the contract, I can expect a definite type of punishment coming from the external world. Both parties know what to expect and usually remember why they expect it.

It is apt to be different with unlimited contracts. The child who promises always to tell the truth may have forgotten this promise when he has grown up. He continues however to feel very guilty if he breaks his promise – fearing of course the punishment which it was agreed was just for the breaking of the promise. The very terms of the contract may also be forgotten, but if the contract is broken, a feeling of uneasiness results. This leads on to the question of the unconscious sense of guilt. Of course unlimited contracts are not always forgotten. For instance, an individual may remember signing a strict temperance pledge as a child, but when grown up realise that it had been made under duress and consequently recognises it could be considered null and void.

The general types of contract can conveniently be tabulated in the following way.

I. VOLUNTARY
   If broken the sense of guilt is realistic.

   (A) *Limited*
       The ordinary legal contract.
   (B) *Unlimited*
       Not often given because of its implications. The commonest is in marriage when a person promises to love and promote the interests of another person in return for similar advantages.

II. IMPOSED
    If broken, the sense of guilt is unrealistic.

   (A) *Limited*
       The reparations clauses of the Versailles treaty are of this order.
   (B) *Unlimited*
       The territorial clauses of the treaty. When given by a person commonly become an ideal.

It will now be interesting to consider some of the contracts which have important psychological consequences.

Voluntary contracts

There is little to be said about the voluntary limited contract. It appears to me to be the basis of morality and its value is so unquestionable and its nature so easily understood that it need cause few emotional difficulties. If all contracts were of this kind, there would I believe be far fewer problems in the world.

The voluntary but unlimited contract has such serious consequences that there are few occasions when it is used. One can only make a contract sensibly when one knows all the facts of the case. One does not sign the lease of a house until one has made quite certain what signature entails. If we are wise we get a solicitor to examine the legal provisions and a surveyor to inspect the house to make quite sure that it is in order. Only then can a sensible decision be arrived at. Unlimited contracts are so apt to contain unknown elements that they are bound to be dangerous. Marriage, which is probably the commonest example, in modern times is a case in point. It is only too frequently entered into without sufficient knowledge and for those people who take the marriage vows seriously may lead to a great conflict of feeling. Of course the marriage oath is very explicit in this matter of knowledge. The difficulties and inconveniences are specifically mentioned "in sickness and in health". In such a promise, an honest attempt is made to impress the implication upon us.

The law takes these questions into consideration. Just as an imposed contract is not legal, so is a promise made without full knowledge of its implications. Now we are not really concerned with the ultimate rights and wrongs of such contracts. It suffices to show that there is a conflict, not only between different people, but also within the individual. A philosopher, a lawyer and a bishop might all given different opinions about the validity of limitless contracts. Different parts of a patient's mind are apt to do the same. Just as the philosopher, a lawyer and a bishop have different standards of right and wrong, so does the individual have different standards contained within him or her and therein lies rich ground for the development of conflict.

Although the theoretical distinction between limited and limitless contracts is clear enough, in practice it is apt to be blurred. "Always" may mean until manhood to the mother, to the small boy it might mean literally forever, since the child takes things very literally. Such a confusion is even more likely to occur over the precise area covered by a promise. For a child of five the promise "always" to be good could include, amongst other things, obeying parents and those in authority and refraining from sexual activity. But most mothers do not want their children to be "good" in this sense forever. Obedience is less important when the boy has become a man, whilst sexual activity should be permissible under certain circumstances. The child however would hardly realise that the mother had these modifications in mind and might easily feel bound by the implicit terms of the original promise.

Such confusions occur very frequently I believe, and are of great importance. But a confusion which is far more subtle and sinister in its results is that which results when a contract is neither imposed nor voluntary, but occupies an ill defined, purposely obscured borderland between the two. Freud with characteristic genius recognised this as the crux of the matter, and built his theory of guilt upon it. Consequently his theory of guilt is, in my opinion, too limited, but since it takes into account one of the most important *practical* problems, it has proved of great value. Before considering this borderland, we will discuss imposed contracts in a little more detail.

Imposed contracts

It is always in the interests of the parents to get the children to make promises to be good. If the child does not promise, the parent's punishment is simply private revenge and is felt as such by him. But if the child can be persuaded to promise to be good, he has undertaken a solemn contract. Now if he breaks this contract, the parent has the *right* to punish the child. The whole principle of the sanctity of treaties is at stake and the parent has perfectly just ground for moral indignation.

We shall do well to consider how such contracts are made. As we have seen, there are two kinds of contract, that which is voluntarily undertaken, and that which is imposed. Now the parent–child relation is peculiarly susceptible to the creation of imposed contracts. For the parent is always the stronger, like the Allies in 1918, and can always dictate terms to the child. Just as the Allies threatened to march on Berlin if the Treaty of Versailles was not signed, so does the parent threaten the child if he will not promise to be good and do whatever he is told. What in fact are the threats which a parent uses? Broadly speaking they are two modes of intimidating the child:

(1) By threatening to use physical violence if the child does not promise.
(2) By threatening to withdraw affection.

Physical violence, of course, presupposes a withdrawal of affection, but only on a limited scale, and lasting for a limited time. But when a parent says "I won't love you unless you promise to be good" the threat is on a far more alarming scale. To the child it may mean that the parent will *never* love him or her again and consequently all the attention and affection, food, lodging and comforts of life are in jeopardy. The possibility of death itself is not so very far away.

This threat therefore is utterly terrifying to a child and consequently extremely effective. Moreover parents feel quite justified in using it. Why should I give care and affection to my child if it won't do what I ask in return, is the parent's feeling. This is not a promise extracted at pistol point but a fair bargain, they would say. Yet from the child's point of view it could be argued that the threat is tantamount to a threat of neglect and death and therefore is equivalent to the beating, and consequently unfair and unjust.

Whatever the morality, it is clear that the child is in a very difficult position. In order to preserve its life it has got to give an undertaking to behave in a way which may put very serious limitations on its enjoyment of life. Consequently it may put a serious strain upon the personality.

Modes of imposing contracts are very numerous, besides these crude ways. For instance some people put others in heavy debt to them simply by showering presents upon them. Such attentions are very often paid by parents to their children and of course often by lovers to their sweethearts, the object being to get something back in return. I am not arguing that genuine altruism is impossible but that altruism is sometimes cover for putting the other under an obligation to give something back. Commonly people sense the meaning of such favours and, should they accept them, do in fact feel under heavy obligation to carry out the contract which they know was implied when they accepted.

Putting children "upon their honour" is a special variety of this. It assumes that the children are already under an obligation to love and obey their parents (or teachers). If the obligation has been voluntarily entered into, there is no reason why it should not be appealed to. Thus if I have voluntarily promised to do some work for a friend during a certain period, he is quite entitled to remind me of this promise, saying that he is trusting my sense of honour to discharge the obligation. When a teacher leaves the room, she reminds her pupils that they have promised to be good and obey her and she will expect that promise to be honoured. But unlike the instance given above the children may have actually entered into no voluntary agreement to obey her, though in a subtle way they have usually had such an obligation imposed upon them. In the great majority of cases, putting children "upon their honour" assumes an obligation which has been imposed upon them.

Freud's ambivalence theory of guilt – anxiety

At the beginning of this paper it was pointed out that Freud's later formulation of his theory of guilt was that it was the expression of the conflict of ambivalence, the fear of destroying that which one loves. It seems to me that *the emotion of love may include an implicit contract.*

We may say that we "love" oysters, meaning that they will give us much instinctual satisfaction. But normally we feel under no obligation to them and we feel no guilt after we have eaten them up, though the story of the *Walrus and the Carpenter* reminds us that unconscious feelings of this sort are not so very far away. These two heroes thought of their oysters as people and it is of course when we love people that we feel guilty when we have destroyed them, or wish to do so. The Walrus and Carpenter were under an obligation to their oysters; they express their affection for them and cruelly mislead them, the oysters trusting in their good faith, and they felt very, very guilty about it. This is what commonly happens in human relationships. One person allows another to rely on his affection and care and an implicit contract grows up that each will always cherish and help the other. How much help and for how long is never clear in an obligation of this sort, but usually a very great deal of both is understood. Now should hatred for any reason arise between the two, the contract to love is automatically broken and guilt is experienced. Such a condition constantly arises in an ambivalent relation and causes continuous and acute conflict.

But apart from love relations which involve vague but far reaching contracts, there is the old problem of not being able to eat one's cake and have it too. Here, I believe, we can begin to draw a distinction between guilt and anxiety, though I propose to deal with this in greater detail later.

Apart from the guilt which the breaking of a love contract by feelings of hatred will entail, there is always the danger that in a fit of hatred, the loved person may be imagined to be destroyed. The destruction of a loved object may be imagined to occur in a fit of hatred, such as wife-beating or else in a fit of loving – such as eating. This latter point is important. It is easy to understand how hate and aggression may lead to destruction; but it is unexpected that love can lead to the same conclusion. Yet it is possible to destroy food which we love by this means, and since sexual love is often felt in oral terms, especially by women, the *fear* of destroying the sexual object seems real enough, though it cannot in fact be done. *The love itself may be destructive* and be feared for that reason.

We may classify the conflicts arising out of a love relationship as follows.

(A) *Where another human is involved*

    (1) Conflicts arising out of the Paradoxical Nature of Love
        (a) no contract present
           e.g. Baby sucking at breast
           → ANXIETY
        (b) implicit contract present
           e.g. later erotic relation
           → GUILT
    (2) Conflicts arising out of ambivalence involving the possibility of destroying or alienating that which we love

      (a) no contract present
         e.g. Temper in baby against mother
         → ANXIETY
      (b) contract present
         e.g. ambivalent love relation
         → GUILT

(B) *Where no other human is involved*

    (1) Conflicts – Paradoxical nature of love
        e.g. child eating sweets
        → ANXIETY
    (2) Conflicts arising from ambivalence
        e.g. child's temper with its toys
        → ANXIETY

Guilt, Anxiety and Fear

It is now possible to discuss the distinction between guilt and anxiety in detail. There are certain real differences of emotion to be discerned here, I believe, but their naming is largely a matter of terminology. "Guilt" has been used in a comparatively limited sense, and there should be no difficulty in agreeing on its use, but "anxiety" has been used very widely and consequently there may be some objection to limiting its use unduly.

The conclusion so far reached has been that guilt is only experienced when an obligation has been undertaken. If we fail in our obligation we know that certain results detrimental to ourselves will follow. This explains partly why guilt has a peculiarly paralysing and isolating effect. Whatever private sins others may sympathise with us for, no mercy can be expected when we have deliberately done what we previously agreed not to do. We anticipate that we can expect protection from no one. It is oneself against the world and so it is not worth trying to escape the results. The great relief which comes when we find someone else shares our guilt is to be explained upon this theory.

What we fear when we feel guilty is punishment and disadvantage. Its peculiar quality is derived from an external source, namely the expectation that we shall receive no help or sympathy and also from an internal source. When we do something which we have promised not to do, it is clear there must be *internal dissension*. The discussion of this I propose to leave for another time, when a systematic analysis of the super-ego might be undertaken.[1]

---

1 [Editors' note:] It would not appear that Bowlby directly undertook a study of internal dissention and the super-ego specifically. His major remarks from the period on the super-ego are contained as Chapter 5 in the present volume.

Now there are other occasions when we may fear the results of our actions, but in which no obligation or contract has been entered into. This is clearest when a state of war exists between people or nations. We may fear the reprisals which our attacks will call forth but no guilt need be experienced unless we have promised always to love all our fellow men. Again a child who is accused unjustly and threatened with punishment may feel great anxiety but will feel the reverse of guilt. Indeed, the child will expect to be able to gain allies – there is no general reason why he should not - whilst there is no internal disagreement. He is quite certain that punishment is wrong and he is prepared to defend himself accordingly.

I propose to use the term *"fear"* for these feelings. Whenever our lives and welfare are threatened, fear is felt. We fear a madman driving a car, we fear earthquakes, we fear the threats of a bully, but we do not feel guilty.

The distinction between guilt and fear is a simple one. To what situations is the term *anxiety* applicable? There are two very different circumstances in which apprehension is felt to which it is often applied.

(1) When there is a conflict in the self without any contract being felt. When a child loses its temper with its mother it finds itself in a predicament. It is furiously angry with its mother, perhaps with good reason, and so it wants to destroy her. But at the same time it is afraid of what will happen to itself as a result. It might hurt its mother or she might think him so hateful that she would abandon him. It is a case of killing the goose who lays the golden eggs. A similar situation, though far less acute arises when a child gets angry with its toys, though this is complicated usually by the displacement of anger from parents. Moreover the danger of eating and so destroying arouses a similar conflict of interests.The term "anxiety" is commonly used to describe these situations, and I propose to retain it.

(2) Sometimes a patient may be terrified of something impersonal like thunder. Yet his terror is far too great to be accounted for by realistic apprehension of danger. There is no broken contract with the sky involved. Yet in such cases it is commonly found that intense guilt is really present, but that instead of fearing just punishment from God against which no protection could be expected, the danger has been displaced to the thunder, from which it is possible to "hide" by getting under the table and also to get others sympathy and help in combating.

The super-ego, guilt and anxiety

The safety of the organism is preserved by a great variety of actions, suited to a number of different dangers. The chief dangers in which we are exposed can be conveniently grouped under the following two headings:

1. dangers from the actions of other people.
2. dangers arising from the non-human world of animals, plants and other natural forces.

Although for descriptive purposes these two groups are clearly defined, in the minds of most people they are much confused.

Now what is it that leads men, both savage and civilised, to expect trouble where none exists or is likely to exist? The employee who is acutely anxious when sent for by the manager who has always been kind and considerate on previous occasions is a case in point. Realistically he may have grounds for expecting a rise in salary, but something in him leads him to anticipate danger. Psycho-analysis speaks of the anxiety which the employee suffers as emanating from his super-ego, and has shown that the reason why danger has been apprehended is due to beliefs held over from childhood as to the nature of other people. During childhood people have come to fear that parents will behave towards themselves in the same savage way that they had wished to behave towards their parents. Such expectations, though quite false, are for various reasons never corrected and come to persist in the mind along with later and more realistic beliefs. Consequently two standards (at least) of the expected behaviour of other people come to be held. For the sake of simplicity I propose calling the one standard "infantile", the other "realistic", though of course the adult standards only approximate to realism.

Now these standards or theories of how others are to be expected to behave are used by the self to further its various ends. On the one hand action designed to satisfy the libido is modified by such standards, which may be quite unduly high or low, on the other self-preservative action is considerably influenced by them, often necessitating heroic efforts to avoid dangers which are in fact non-existent.

If two different standards or theories about what can be expected obtain simultaneously a conflict will ensue. Thus a patient may realistically believe that the analyst is trying to help him, but his infantile theories may tell him that all people are planning to spy out his faults and punish him. A conflict ensues as to whether to continue going to the analyst or keep clear of him. Such concerns raise the question of how the infantile theories are arrived at in childhood and why they should persist into adult life.

Construction of infantile theories

Our chief reason for expecting people to behave in a particular way is because we have observed them behave thus previously. Each individual has idiosyncrasies and we get to know them after a while and act accordingly. Children are very quick to observe how others will behave and they rapidly acquire working rules not only as to how all human beings behave, but also how individuals behave. What concerns us chiefly is how people will behave towards ourselves. A small girl may learn that provided she behaves in a certain way, she can be sure of the attentions of her father. She may also learn to expect jealousy from her mother. Such expectations are not necessarily consciously worked out but arrived at in just the same direct way that we know that water will be wet. But one of the chief faults of the human mind is to generalise from insufficient data. This generalisation is simply a primitive type of scientific theory and that is why I have used the term "theory" for this class of expectation, rather than "phantasy" which suggests little or no connection with reality.

People do not modify their theories easily. It is rare to find people who have minds which can be influenced. The tenacity with which humans hold to their generalisations, whether primitive and infantile or comparatively adult and realistic, is one of our most striking characteristics. Quite apart therefore from factors such as repression it must be realised that a generalisation once arrived at is not likely to be changed except by a long and slow process. When however some of these theories are repressed, and the fruits of new experience cannot be related to them, no modification at all is to be expected.

Before proceeding to inquire why these theories should be insulated from new experience – repressed – two other methods of arriving at such theories are to be noted. For instance other people may *explain* how they may be expected to behave by threatening or tantalising. If you do so and so I will give you a sweet; if you do something else I will give you a beating. Such threats and promises are naturally quickly worked into our theories of people's behaviour.

Then there are contracts, in their multiplicity of forms. If I have promised to be a good boy and my father has promised to thrash me if I'm not, then I have clearly defined grounds for certain expectations. The details of such contracts, as we have seen, may be "forgotten" but they have often been worked into our "unconscious" theories and continue to influence our expectations long after they were supposed to expire.

As an example of the latter two ways of arriving at expectations, a recent case comes to my mind. A girl had been brought up very strictly never to criticise and complain about her parents. She had partially accepted this and promised to keep it in order to retain her mother's affection, but it was maintained I think purely under the threat of punishment. She had in fact much to complain about, for she was treated as a drudge by all members of the family and her mother demanded her constant presence so that she could not go out and enjoy herself. But to complain would have meant landing herself in the danger which her mother's threats and her own promises had given her good reason to expect. These expectations held good even after her mother's death and there was good evidence to show that she still expected the return of her mother from the grave to punish her if she expressed the bitter complaints which she had in her heart.

This patient also suggests a fourth and very important way in which infantile theories come to be formed. Our knowledge of other people is largely founded upon our knowledge of ourselves. Children therefore may come to expect that adults will be fully as greedy and angry as they know they themselves can be. The patient whom I have just described not only expected "reasonable" punishment from her mother, but feared, amongst other things. that she would die of cancer like her mother and be stabbed in the back by me, both the result of expecting an exact retaliatory punishment.

The four ways in which we learn to account for other people's behaviour towards ourselves can be listed as different groups of expectations:

Group 1)   Expectations based upon general observation
Group 2)   Expectations based upon specific threats and promises
Group 3)   Expectations based upon an agreed contract
Group 4)   Expectations based upon knowledge of our own feelings and wishes

The resulting theories are far less general propositions as to how people behave amongst themselves than specific prophecies as to how they will behave towards *ourselves* in certain specific circumstances which we may produce. We are concerned to know what mother will do if we lose our temper and what nurse will do if we hit the baby. If our theories tell us to expect punishment if we do either of these, then we become anxious if we feel a wish to do either. Our expectations of other people's actions from moment to moment will also depend then on our own wishes at the given moment, and our confidence in our own ability to control those wishes.

This confidence in controlling our own wishes is of very great importance. It is clear that if we can control our actions, no anxiety need be felt, because we should refrain from hitting the baby if people were about and likely to discover. The inability to control wishes results particularly from repression. A wish is felt to be so dangerous and morally bad (i.e. conflicting with contracts) that peace of mind is only obtained by pretending we don't feel it at all. By ignoring it, we deliberately refuse to have anything more to do with it and consequently have no control over it.

The exact conditions under which repression occurs need investigation. It is possible, I think, that it is always the result of *moral* disapproval.

To return to a consideration of actions apart from wishes. It is clear that our actual behaviour will be based upon our theories, and it will be appropriate or inappropriate just in so far as our theories are accurate or not. Moreover, in order not to have to think everything out afresh each time, *rules of conduct* will emerge from these theories which will be the common and unthinking response of the organism to situations. These rules of conduct remind us of the three types of ego-ideal:

Type A) Those voluntarily chosen either in childhood or later life as general rules of that behaviour which will lead to greatest happiness (includes some of group 1 and 2).

Type B) Ideals which have been adopted against our conscious will and in the face of duress and about which we have made no promise (group 2).

Type C) Ideals which form part of a contract entered into either voluntarily or involuntarily, one part of the contract being of an eternal character.

It will now be seen that the rules under ego-ideals of Type A) are likely to be founded upon the theories in Group 1), that is expectations based upon common observation. Rules under ego-ideals of Type B) follow from the theories in Group 2). And that those of Type C) follow from those in Group 3). All the ideals will be influenced by processes from Group 4), the attribution of our own feelings to other people.

The opportunity of conflict between these different codes of conduct is enormous, for not only have we the persistence of infantile theories and rules of conduct alongside more adult ones, but there is a likelihood of the ideals from Group A conflicting with those in Group B or C. It is true that there *need* be no conflict between them, for Group A) could include everything. If we know that we are fined for driving more than thirty miles per hour in Oxford, we can either decide to break the law and take the consequences or keep it.

The wise man undertakes no obligations which he knows may be difficult or impossible to discharge, in other words, he will avoid obligations which conflict with his general rules of behaviour. An example of a particularly difficult obligation to decide about is in the case of a daughter who has always looked after her mother, but who later wants to get married. Such a situation is notoriously difficult but in no sense insoluble. The upshot is this. If the various rules of conduct and theories of other people behaviour can be weighed against each other dilemmas can be solved or negotiated. When for various reasons they are divorced, and the existence of one denied by the conscious mind, their differing counsels conflict more absolutely and destructively. Our next concern is to know why two rules of personal conduct or two theories about other peoples' behaviour should be so divorced.

Separation of infantile theories from adult theories

One thing is immediately evident – the enormous advantage which we all get from "forgetting" obligations. If we genuinely forgot an obligation, some sympathy would be extended to us; it would not be regarded as so deliberately bad. An alternative is, whilst admitting the obligation, to deny that we broke it. I remember being lent a clockwork engine by my brother, when I was about eight. In receiving the loan, we assumed I had promised to treat it carefully and to take responsibility if it got broken. While he was away I experimented with it, and broke it. But considering the matter I managed to convince myself that it was a very poor engine. This piece of self-deception succeeded sufficiently for me to convince my brother and mother that the engine had "come to pieces in my hands".

When we can excuse ourselves, we often do. To forget the incident altogether rids us of these doubts. So we think. Analytic experience goes to show however that uncertainty remains and guilt continues despite the incident being forgotten. Really we broke the obligation deliberately and perhaps this will be found out, perhaps punishment will come later – at the last judgement if not before. Our expectation of how others will behave towards us is seriously affected by such hidden minor sins, the memory of which may be repressed.

Repression can be arrived at in various ways:

1. We can deny all knowledge of having involved ourselves in an obligation.
2. We can deny any occasion when we broke one.
3. We can deny any feeling or wish to break one e.g. hatred.
4. We can deny any feeling or wish which could involve us in one e.g. libidinal wishes.

All these can be denied, forgotten, and the conscious mind relieved consequently of guilt and fear of punishment. We were not guilty, we can say, with some degree of honesty. Punishment is unfair, allies must be found to protect us.

Repression however is often inadequate. Sometimes all feeling has gone, but a patient's actions are such that they can only be explained by supposing that he has felt guilty in the past and only avoids it by acts of reparation which we now see him making. Other patients fear all manner of dangers and this again can be explained by supposing that they are constantly fearing punishment. Patients such as these are said to have an unconscious sense of guilt.

It is in this way that two standards of how people may be expected to behave come to be held simultaneously. We feel guilt and fear punishment, but both of these we deny. Infantile theories and rules of conduct persist together with more adult ones. The process of repression has kept them apart, no checking has been allowed to go on and so despite the antiquity of the infantile it continues to affect conduct in various ways.

Ego and super-ego

The terms ego and super-ego have been introduced to describe these different types of organisation. The term ego is used to describe our conscious, adult and comparatively realistic theories of people's behaviour and the power that guides our deliberate actions based upon these theories. Broadly speaking, therefore, it corresponds to Group 1) theories and Type A) ego-ideals. What I have included in Type A) ego-ideals is complicated by the process of identification, but it seems to me that, in so far as these ideals are voluntarily adopted and relate so closely to consciousness that despite the term, ego-ideal, they must be included under the ego. The distinction between long-run ego-interests and short-run ego-interests is one only of degree, for these can be and are closely organised together in "normal" people. Consequently it is convenient to use the same term to cover the organisation which controls them.

The term super-ego has been used rather obscurely. Freud uses it to cover the organisation which promotes

1. Long-run ego interests (ego-ideals).
2. Our feelings of obligation to people (conscience).
3. Our feelings of remorse when we have broken our obligations.
4. Our tendency to punish ourselves when we have sinned.

Before proceeding with theories of its origin, I want to draw attention to the way in which the term is at present used. James Strachey in his recent paper "The Nature of the Therapeutic Action in Psycho-Analysis" (Strachey, 1934) discusses the modifications which he believes the super-ego undergoes during treatment. He does not define or describe the term, but what he seems to me to mean throughout and consistently is simply a person's infantile theories of what other people are like and how he ought to behave in order to get along in the world (preserve himself and get libidinal satisfaction). In effect what Strachey holds is that in analysis these infantile theories, which are mostly unconscious, are brought to the light of day and re-examined and consequently modified. Mrs Klein's use of the term is I think the same as Strachey's.

The identification of the super-ego with the infantile theories seems to me most illuminating. It is, I think, a better description than Freud's own. The distinction between infantile theories and adult theories is one which, if not always easy to detect in practice, is at least a clear theoretical distinction. Its chief advantage seems to me to be that it distinguishes between infantile and adult ego-ideals and conscience. Freud did not make this distinction and consequently grouped them all together under the heading super-ego. Much of such a super-ego is infantile but some of course is realistic and though Freud realised that there was this difficulty, I don't think he has ever seen it very clearly.

The grouping which Strachey's paper seems to me to propose distinguishes between infantile conscience and adult conscience. The latter it apportions to the ego, because as discussed previously, in a well-organised personality the ego can voluntarily undertake obligations and is its own conscience.

<u>Adult and Realistic</u>

SHORT-RUN EGO-INTERESTS	LONG-RUN EGO-INTERESTS = EGO-IDEAL
WISHES	SENSE OF CONTRACTS

<u>Dating from Infancy</u>

SHORT-RUN EGO-INTERESTS	LONG-RUN EGO-INTERESTS = EGO-IDEAL
WISHES	SENSE OF CONTRACTS

A schematic presentation may help.

The right hand column includes those parts of the mind which Freud calls super-ego. Those in the second row are what I propose to call super-ego and are what I believe actually are meant by Strachey and Mrs Klein.

I do not propose to examine Freud's theories in detail now, because I find them extremely difficult to follow and understand. But we must note further attributes of the super-ego which seem to me more in the nature of inferences than actual observation. Freud accounts for the origin of conscience and ego-ideals by supposing that the ego makes certain strong and important identifications with the parents.

"If they obtain the upper hand and become too numerous, unduly intense and incompatible with one another, a pathological outcome will not be far off."

He writes of the origin of the ego-ideal: "behind the ego-ideal lies hidden the first and most important identification of all, the identification with the father", (Freud, 1923b, p.38).

Mrs Klein of course has done a lot of work on this topic which will need close examination.

Problem of identification

What I have previously written goes to indicate what my theories regarding origin of super-ego are likely to be.

The upshot of my argument is that the functions of the super-ego are no different from those of the ego. These may be described as

1) To store up data as to how other people are towards the self, thereby indicating how they may be expected to behave in the future.
2) To decide upon and carry out actions which will promote the libidinal ends and preserve the self from danger (especially from other people). This it does

    (a) by inhibiting certain wishes (id wishes) which would lead the person into danger

    (b) by promoting other actions which will further these ends. (ego-ideals - undertaking contracts, etc)

The only difference, I think, between the ego and the super-ego is that the super-ego is working with an archaic set of data, whilst the ego is comparatively up-to-date. Serious conflict comes when these two differ and one is as strong as the other.

Self-punishment

The phenomenon of self-punishment was one of the first observations to draw Freud's attention to a property in the ego beyond those we ordinarily know. His theory of the super-ego is very intimately bound up with observation upon self-punishment and no modification of super-ego theory can be considered which will not account for it.

Freud's own account is to be found both in *Civilisation and its Discontents,* (Freud, 1930a) and also in the *New Introductory Lectures on Psycho-Analysis,* (Freud, 1933a).

"This unconscious need for punishment.... will correspond to a piece of aggressiveness which has been internalised and taken over by the super-ego" (Freud, 1933a, p.141). Because of the child's love fixation upon its parents, no aggressiveness can be directed against them. The aggressiveness is then "taken over" by the super-ego and directed against the ego.

It is easy to understand the child's fear and dislike of expressing its aggression upon its parents. In order to prevent aggression being vented, part of the ego must be set apart to deal with it (It is the ego's function to deal sensibly with id-impulses by organising them, slowing them up and re-directing them as circumstances recognise. In dealing with the aggression stimulated by parents, it is only doing its usual job). This particular part of the ego Freud terms the super-ego. What does it do with these embarrassing aggressions? It might direct them to persons other than parents or it might inhibit them altogether (if that is possible). What Freud maintains that it does, at any rate sometimes, is to introject them – i.e. to direct them against the ego itself. The super-ego from then on "exercises the same propensity to harsh aggressiveness against the ego that the ego would have liked to enjoy against others". (Freud, 1930a, p.105). In other words one part of the ego, whose special duty it is to organise these aggressive impulses, finds the best way of doing this is by venting it upon the self.

This is clear and understandable, but it does not explain why it should be felt as self-*punishment,* rather than self-mutilation. The moral element needs explanation and this Freud gives by saying that guilt is always experienced when ambivalent feelings are present. Consequently this "introjection" of aggression not only avoids feelings of guilt by resolving the ambivalence, but actually punishes the guilty party.

I am inclined to think that the situation is more complicated. I have given my reasons for wishing to modify Freud's theory of guilt. The mere presence of ambivalence is not enough to produce guilt. A promise of some sort is also necessary. Punishment moreover supports something more purposeful than the turning of aggression upon the self simply because there is nowhere else to expend it. Why is the aggression not turned upon other outsiders when they are present? Why must it always be upon the self?

Three elements in this process of self-punishment must, I think, be distinguished. They are very commonly blended I suspect and Freud, as usual, has struck upon the common and important clinical manifestation. But a clear theoretical analysis is only possible when these elements are considered separately.

Firstly there is much evidence to show that the aggressive impulse, like the sexual, will take any object for its expression rather than none. If we can't vent our wrath on our employers we vent it upon our servants. The displacement may not be very satisfactory but it is better than nothing. It would not therefore be surprising to find that, when no one else was available, the aggression is expressed upon the self. Anything to express it! Such a theory is interestingly born out by monkeys. Zuckerman (1932) describes how monkeys will mutilate themselves if they are alone in their cages and visitors make them angry. The simplest theory to explain such a happening is displacement of aggression from the original object to the only other present, namely the self.

Now humans are rarely in iron cages. They always have others to vent this wrath on, so why do they ever choose themselves? *Although not in iron-cages, humans are often in cages of inhibition.* They *feel* that any overt manifestation of aggression against anyone will be met by universal revenge. (This is the result of infantile theories). Consequently it is too dangerous to attack others and the only object left is the self. This factor is rarely present alone, but explains the fierceness of the attacks which some people launch upon themselves.

A second element is, of course, the simple desire to hurt those who one wishes to hurt, but which inhibitions protect from overt attack. "They will be very sorry when I'm dead". This indirect attack upon others is also carried out in another way. If a patient feels that they have got their foe within them (introjected them) then an attack upon the self is also an attack upon the introjected enemy.

The third element is the moral element. When a person is feeling terribly guilty he wants to be punished to get it over and done with. There is nothing which is so *exhausting* as the waiting for punishment to be delivered when we have reason to expect it. We want to know the worst, largely because our infantile theories lead us to expect punishments of shocking severity and we know (that is our adult theories tell us) that nothing in reality will be as bad as that. As long as a child has done wrong and is awaiting punishment, he cannot expect his parents love. As soon as the beating is over, most parents will regard the incident as over and done with. The child is loved once more. Again how much preferable is a finite misfortune, such as physical hurt or even financial loss, to the endless punishment which not being loved entails. No punishment is more serious or frightening for a child than being told by its parents that they no longer love it. Again immediate punishment, however severe is preferable; this again leads the culprit to take the punishment with his own hands.

The neurotic or psychotic constantly expects punishment for sins which he either really committed and wanted to commit when he was quite small. Feelings of hatred and aggression are regarded with horror by his infantile theories since they are held to break numerous contracts. But these feelings are sometimes evoked and acute feelings of guilt result. A patient of mine showed this very clearly. He was a young man of about twenty five who had been walking out with a girl for some years. Due partly to perceptions that she was flirting with other men in his office, he began to get impulses to hurt her. He became severely depressed and had considerable overt guilt about these impulses. At one interview he asked me whether I thought it would do him good if a friend of his – a heavy-weight boxer – were to knock him out. Clearly he felt it might and he was deliberately soliciting punishment for what he felt to be very wicked impulses. This man felt, I suspect, that death alone would atone for his terrible feelings. But he hoped that being knocked out might do instead. When we are hurt people are less cruel as a rule and we can expect punishments to be mitigated.

Although a serious study of suicide must strictly be clinical, it is worthwhile pointing out the three mechanisms which come into play and the type of suicide likely to be committed.

1) A simple attack upon the self because internal inhibitions prevent overt attack.
2) An attack upon the self which is aimed at the internalised object. Both these methods are likely to be violent and active attacks, such as shooting or throat-cutting.
3) A self-sacrifice. A feeling that only by death itself can the love of the important people be regained. This is likely to be more passive and especially liable to invite another person to do the damage, as happens when a person throws themselves under a train.

Of course all these factors are commonly intermixed, but I suspect that one or another is usually predominant.

References

Freud, S. (1923b). *The Ego and the Id. S. E., 19*: 3–66. London: Hogarth Press.
Freud, S. (1930a). *Civilisation and its Discontents. S. E., 21*: 59–145. London: Hogarth Press.

Freud, S. (1933a). *New Introductory Lectures on Psycho-Analysis. S. E., 22*: 3–182. London: Hogarth Press.

Strachey, J. (1934). The nature of the therapeutic action in psycho-analysis. *International Journal of Psycho-Analysis, 15*: 127–159.

Zuckerman, S. (1932). *The Social Life of Monkeys and Apes*. London: Routledge.

Part 3

Seminars at Stanford and the Tavistock

Chapter 8

A psycho-analytic approach to conflict and its regulation

A seminar delivered to members of the Stanford Conflict Seminar, January, 1958

[Editors: Wellcome Collection Archive PP/BOW/H.67]

From: John Bowlby
To: Members of Conflict Seminar.

The attached notes are circulated before the meeting on Friday 10th January and are intended as an indication of how I hope to discuss my theme.

1. My plan will be briefly to recapitulate certain points from the case of Mrs. K.[1] which I presented in November. These are:

   (a) her principal problems centred on her intense conflict of ambivalence towards her mother,

   (b) her illness resulted from the unfavourable modes which she had adopted for regulating the conflict,

   (c) her progress in treatment was due to her being enabled to adopt more favourable methods of regulation.

2. This case illustrates the main points of my thesis which are:

   I. Intrapsychic conflict is inevitable and ubiquitous.

   II. A major criterion for assessing the state of mental health of a personality lies in the modes of regulating intrapsychic conflicts characteristic of that personality. From these propositions it follows that:

   III. A major area for preventing the development of mental ill-health lies in so treating children that they are enabled as they develop to adopt more favourable methods of conflict regulation.

---

1 [Editors' note:] No record has been found of the November presentation. The description is relatively generic – it could fit many patients. However, it also sounds like Bowlby's account of Mrs Q., the most frequently discussed of Bowlby's patients. The first published mention is in: Bowlby, J. (1963).

IV.   A chief task of treatment is to help the patient acquire better methods of regulating intrapsychic conflict than he hitherto had available.

I hope to say a little about each of these points.

Point I. Intrapsychic conflict is inevitable and ubiquitous.

3.   I shall indicate briefly its place in the history of psychoanalytic theory and practice.
4.   I shall make a comparison with the point of view expressed by Ralph Dahrendorf[2] with which I am in close agreement. In Section VII of his first memo, he summarised his views thus:

"Our main objective in these notes is the exploration of some of the principles underlying the regulation of interest group conflict. On the basis of the preceding considerations we can now tentatively offer some generalizations:

1)   Social conflict is universal in the sense that wherever there are social organizations with an authority structure there are causes for conflict.
2)   Regulation of conflict can apply only to the regulation of the expressions, not the causes of conflict.
3)   Resolution of conflict in the sense of its ultimate abolition is not realistically possible.
4)   Suppression of conflict in the sense of its ultimate abolition is not realistically possible."

5.   It seems to me probable that wherever there is differentiation within a system (irrespective of the kind of system) there is bound to be intra-systemic conflict. I therefore suspect that sociologists and psychoanalysts are dealing with similar problems in dissimilar systems.
6.   As regards Dahrendorf's second point, I have a criticism. It seems to me sensible always to consider ways by which the causes of any particular conflict may be altered so that the conflict is made more manageable, *provided always* that we recognise that some degree of conflict is inevitable. I believe therefore that there are always two tasks:

(a)   to consider the practicability and desirability of taking action to alter the causes of conflict.
(b)   to take steps for improving modes of regulating it.

2 [Editors' note:] Ralph Dahrendorf was a fellow with Bowlby during 1957-58 at the Centre for Advanced Study, Stanford. Dahrendorf (1959) *Class and Class Conflict in Industrial Society.*

As Dahrendorf emphasises, too much attention is usually given to the first and too little to the second of these.

Point II. A major criterion for assessing the state of mental health of a personality lies in the modes of regulating intrapsychic conflict characteristic of that personality.

7. As in all matters of health and illness here we come to value judgments. I suspect that the criteria for judging modes of regulating intrapsychic conflict as better or worse will be found along these lines

    (a) the extent to which the personality is able on balance to maximise its satisfactions,
    (b) the extent to which the personality is able to preserve its functioning intact in conditions of emotional stress.

8. Provided we are concerned only with gross differentiation, criterion (a) is fairly easy to use: those who, because of inhibitions or a tendency to self-frustrating actions, are unable to achieve reasonable satisfactions are classed as unhealthy. On the other hand, once a reasonable degree of satisfaction is obtainable by the personality, it is not possible to use this criterion effectively, since we have no refined methods of measuring or comparing satisfactions.

9. Criterion (b) also has the limitation that it is difficult to predict the extent to which a personality will remain intact in conditions of emotional stress in the absence of such stress. However, it is reasonable to hope we may gradually improve our skills in the application of both criteria.

10. There is clearly an empirical task of discovering which modes of regulating conflict meet these criteria. Much clinical evidence from psychoanalysis suggests that, on balance, modes which attempt the suppression of conflict are unsatisfactory and that modes which give it full recognition are better. This again reminds us of Dahrendorf's views:

    1) Conflict can be effectively regulated only if those involved recognise the universality of conflict. This indicates a value premise of effective regulation, and one that departs from the values prevalent in many industrial societies today. It might be argued that non-acceptance of conflict as an element of social life is in fact one of the main causes for the failure of many societies and social organizations to regulate conflict successfully.

Point III. A major area for preventing the development of mental ill health lies in so treating children that they are enabled as they develop to adopt more favourable methods of conflict regulation.

11. This is the theme of the lecture I gave at the time of the Freud Centenary, the bulk of which was incorporated and circulated before the first occasion I spoke to the seminar, under the title "A psycho-analytic view of conflict and its regulation". In it I described two classes of conditions which make for difficulty:

    (a) experiences such as mother-child separation or parental rejection, which seem to have the effect of greatly intensifying both components of ambivalence,

    (b) parental attitudes, conscious or unconscious, which in effect forbid the child to express or ever entertain hostile feelings towards the parents.

The processes set up by these two classes of conditions are probably rather different, although I have yet to get around to studying them systematically and can only indicate briefly what I think they may be.

12. The latter case is probably the easier to consider first, though even here many different processes may be involved. For instance, parental attitudes may lead to

    (a) the guilt which we all feel when we are angry or unkind to those we love becoming maximised,

    (b) the anxiety we all feel in similar circumstances that the loved person will be either damaged or alienated becoming maximised (Cf. the case of Mrs. K.),

    (c) punishment being used in such a way that the child is afraid of the consequences of any expression or even the entertainment of hostile wishes.

In all these cases the child may gradually develop a state of mind in which he is genuinely unaware of such wishes.

13. These three methods of child control (and various combinations of them) have in common the belief that conflict between children and parents can be suppressed and that this is desirable. They all three have the effect that the intra-psychic conflict in the child is in different degrees driven underground. In addition to repression of one component of the conflict (usually hate but sometimes love), the child usually resorts to defences such as displacement (cf. Mrs. K.), projection, and others.

14. The processes brought into play when conflict is greatly intensified by, for instance, separation experiences may be rather different, though the result is again a banishment from consciousness of one or other or both components of the conflict. (Psychoanalysis has for long recognised different types of process leading to a splitting off of an impulse from consciousness – e.g., primal and secondary repression,

denial, etc. My impression is that neither terminology nor thinking on this theme are very clear, but I have yet to do systematic reading.)

15.   In trying to understand the nature of these processes I want to explore the relevance of ideas about integration-span being restricted in conditions of stress. For instance, there is much evidence that, while under stress, there is a tendency for the organism to be influenced in its behaviour by fewer determinants than when stress is absent, and I suspect this is true of *both inner and outer determinants of behaviour*. If this is so, there might well be a tendency for an individual who is under persistent and severe stress to continue to restrict the number of determinants which he can permit to operate in respect of each of his actions. The persistent restriction of inner determinants to a few (which is the same as the persistent exclusion of others) may be a clue to the nature of repression.

16.   I picture this restriction of determinants in conditions of stress as an emergency device which, inefficient though it may be in ordinary conditions, may be expedient in conditions of emergency. If this is true it would follow that the healthily functioning personality would vary the number of determinants of action which he permitted according to the conditions he was facing; and a lack of such flexibility would be a sign of ill health.

17.   Clinical experience strongly suggests that during infancy and early childhood there is much plasticity in regard to modes which can be adopted for regulating conflicts, but that those which are adopted tend to stabilise and to persist. Thus it seems likely that there are critical periods in such development.

Point IV. A direct task of treatment is to help the patient acquire better methods of regulating intra-psychic conflict.

18.   Traditionally the process of psychoanalytic therapy has been conceived as "making what is unconscious conscious." Empirically it seems to be true that the more aware an individual is of his own motives, which it is contended are always in some degree incompatible with one another, the more effectively can he regulate the resulting conflicts. This is hardly surprising since only if we are alive to conflicting issues are we likely to take a course of action which maximises satisfaction. Accurate though the traditional description is, I believe that a better description of psychoanalytic therapy is that it seeks to enable the patient to utilise a method of regulating conflict characterised by (a) a clear recognition of the inevitability and ubiquity of intra-psychic conflict and (b) as clear a recognition as possible of the nature of all motivations present at any one time. Once the process of "laying candidly on the table" all active motivations

has become habitual there is of course no need for it thenceforward to be carried out consciously.

19. These characteristics are clearly similar to those which Dahrendorf regards as necessary for the effective regulation of interest group conflict in social organisations, namely conflict is recognised as universal and that "the conflicting groups are formalized identifiable organizations".

If we consider Dahrendorf's table on the role of the third party in the regulation of conflict (see his second memo p. 5), it might be suggested that the role of the psychoanalyst is that of mediator (Role B). His assistance is asked for voluntarily and accepted voluntarily. His task is to help all subsystems within the personality to become aware of the existence and nature of each other, to tolerate one another without too much anxiety and guilt and to live with each other as parts of the total system, namely the personality itself.

References

Bowlby, J. (1963). Pathological mourning and childhood mourning. *Journal of the American Psychoanalytic Association*, *11*: 500–541.

Bowlby, J. (1979). By ethology out of psychoanalysis: An experiment in interbreeding. *Animal Behaviour, 28*: 649–656.

Bowlby, J. (1984). Violence in the family as a disorder of the attachment and caregiving systems. *The American Journal of Psychoanalysis, 44*: 9–27.

Dahrendorf, R. (1959). *Class and Class Conflict in Industrial Society.* Stanford: Stanford University Press.

Chapter 9

A seminar delivered to members of the Stanford Conflict Seminar, February, 1958

[Editors: Wellcome Collection Archive, PP/BOW/H.67]

From: John Bowlby, Ralf Dahrendorf[1]

In order to facilitate discussion in the winding up session(s) of the Conflict Seminar, we have decided to attempt a short summary of earlier discussions, concentrating on the more general aspects involved. In particular, three recurrent sets of problems require attention:

    I.   There are the terminological problems which, it is suggested, are in many ways more than "just terminological".

   II. The point of view implicit or explicit in the papers presented may be submitted to some further scrutiny.

 III. The seminar has been planned as an "interdisciplinary" venture, but we have not yet addressed ourselves directly to the problems inherent in such an approach. The following notes should be thought of as a basis for discussion, and are not intended to prescribe either its course or its outcome.

I.   Terms

Two different notions of *conflict* emerged in the discussions of the seminar, and the difference between them has not always been sufficiently explicit. According to one notion, conflict exists if and only if the peaceful operation of societies, social institutions, social relations and personalities breaks down and gives way to more or less violent expressions of antagonism or ambivalence. Defined in this way, there is conflict in industry during a strike, in the personality during a breakdown, but there is no conflict in "normally functioning" enterprises or personalities. The second notion – advanced above

---

1 [Editors' note:] Ralph Dahrendorf was a fellow with Bowlby during 1957–1958 at the Centre for Advanced Study, Stanford. Dahrendorf (1959) *Class and Class Conflict in Industrial Society.*

all by John Bowlby and Ralf Dahrendorf – speaks of conflict wherever there are antagonisms of interest, purpose or emotion, independent of their expression in overt warfare. Thus, conflict exists in the enterprise or the personality, even if strikes or breakdowns are absent. It will be seen that for the formulation of general propositions about conflict it is of considerable importance which of these definitions is accepted.

There are two dimensions of conflict the distinction of which seems useful. Conflicts can vary in their *intensity*, i.e. in the amount of energy spent by conflicting forces, the importance attached by these forces to certain issues, the "cost" of victory or defeat. Conflicts can also vary in their *violence* of expression, i.e. the militancy of the means chosen for expressing conflict. It is important to distinguish clearly between these two.

By *regulation of conflict* is understood, in the most general sense, any mode of dealing with conflict. Regulation, in this sense, does not imply any value judgment as to its desirability or effectiveness.

[2]*Resolution of conflict* is one form of regulation, namely, regulation designed to do away with the roots of conflict and thereby abolish it altogether. When conflict is resolved in this way, it is not merely settled for a limited period of time, but settled once and for all.

By *suppression of conflict* we understand the deliberate or unconscious attempt to prevent conflicting forces from gaining expression, such as the prohibition of strikes or political opposition, or repression of "emotions" (namely, motivation characterized by strong emotion).

[3]By *conciliation* we mean a mode of conflict regulation which provides institutions or mechanisms for the conflicting parties or forces to "have it out", i.e. to express their conflicting interests, purposes, emotions and arrive at decisions, without any interference by third parties. Conciliation is the autonomous regulation of conflict by the parties involved. It may or may not lead to agreed decisions. (The word "conciliation" has certain unfortunate valuational overtones. If a better term can be found, we should be glad to replace it.)

Mediation, on the other had, is a way of regulating conflict that involves the participation of a third party in a mediating capacity, i.e. without any authority to make binding decisions. The "mediator" in industrial conflict, and the psychoanalyst in personality conflict, acts in this sense as a third party, and attempts to increase communication and mutual understanding.

Arbitration, finally, is a mode of conflict regulation in which a third party is endowed (by the conflicting parties, or by an outside agency) with

---

2 [Editors' note:] Handwritten note on top right corner of the page: "Distraction" and "Redirection".

3 [Editors' note:] Handwritten margin note: "negotiation".

the authority and/or power to make binding decisions about the relative merits of conflicting issues.

By *rules of the game* we understand such norms as present the formal framework of conflict regulation, in so far as these are accepted by conflicting forces. (Norms that operate as rules of the game in one set of conditions may under changed conditions become prejudicial to the case of one of the disputants. This is an empirical problem worthy of further enquiry.)

II.   Propositions

1)   Conflict is ubiquitous. In all differentiated systems, conflict is invariably present.

It is obvious that this statement makes sense only on the basis of the second definition of conflict above; in that sense, it illustrates the importance of terminological decisions. Clearly, ubiquity of conflict cannot mean ubiquity of violent conflict; what is meant here is, rather, that all differentiated systems contain at any point in time tensions and antagonisms which require regulation, and which can result in militant conflict at any time. The expression "differentiated system" is very general. For social organizations, Ralf Dahrendorf has suggested specifying the kind of differentiation in question by concentrating on relations of constraint (authority structure) as characteristics of "systems" in which conflict is ubiquitous.

2)   The intensity of conflict varies according to certain factors like:

a)   the degree of involvement of persons in conflicts.
b)   the degree to which regulation of conflicts is effective.

It is likely that, in the personality, involvement in conflicts increases with the immediacy of relations to which conflict is directed, i.e. ambivalence towards parents is likely to produce more intense conflicts than ambivalence towards colleagues. In social conflict, involvement would appear to be similarly a function of the immediate importance of the social context, i.e. conflict in industry, where people earn their living, is more intense than conflict in a chess club.

3)   The violence of expression of conflict varies inversely with the effective regulation of conflict. The better conflict is regulated, the less violent is it likely to be.

4)   Resolution of conflict is not realistically possible. Resolution as defined above means abolition of conflict. It follows from proposition 1 that this is not possible in differentiated systems. Although specific issues of conflict (like a particular wage claim) may be settled once and for all, the conflict giving rise to these issues is thereby not "resolved", but persists. In this sense, all attempts at conflict resolution are ill-advised.

5) Suppression of conflict is not an effective mode of regulation; in the long run it cannot succeed.This proposition, although obvious in some ways, is nevertheless problematic in others, and requires further discussion. Suppression of conflict may have one of several results. It may temporarily silence forbidden emotions or interests, only to let them come up again at a later time with doubled violence. It may also redirect conflicting forces, so that they spring up in unexpected places and produce what some call "unrealistic conflict". In any case, suppression does not effectively settle conflict, but at best delays or distorts its expression.

6) Social policy and psychological therapy, if aiming at a relatively satisfactory operation of social organizations and personalities, require the introduction and regular usage of effective and favourable modes of conflict regulation.This statement clearly implies a value judgment, and one about which disagreement is possible. Thus, it is an open question – particularly in the social sphere – what exactly a "relatively satisfactory operation" implies. It might be suggested that even violent conflict can under some circumstances be desirable to advance social (and personality?) development. In any case, it seems clear that, if we want relatively peaceful and reliable conditions, inherent conflicts will have to be regulated by means other than resolution and suppression.

7) The minimum requirements of successful conflict regulation would seem to be:

    a) recognition of the presence of conflict and of the true nature of conflicting forces,
    b) expression (if necessary, through organizations) of conflicting forces,
    c) establishment of certain rules of the game.

8) In addition to the minimum requirements a number of conditions would appear to be favourable to effective conflict regulation.Among these conditions two have been given special attention in earlier discussions. One was the presence of a mediator who promotes mutual understanding between both parties or forces without imposing his decision upon them. John Bowlby suggested that this was also the role of the analyst. The other condition discussed at some length by Frank Newman is the adherence to some kind of "due process", including, in most cases, a "hearing". Undoubtedly, further conditions could be specified.

9) Modes of regulating conflict will vary in their effectiveness according to the conditions of conflict. One such condition is that of greater or lesser emergency.

The less urgent, the more appropriate it is to take account of many considerations before reaching decisions; the more urgent the better it is to restrict determinants of action. Cf. John Bowlby's notion of the integration-span being restricted in conditions of stress (paragraphs 15 and 16 of note of early January),[4] and Frank Newman's discussion of limitations of "due process" in conditions of emergency.[5]

III.   Problems of interdisciplinary discussions

Interdisciplinary discussions are both tempting and dangerous. To avoid undesirable consequences, it is perhaps best to regulate this conflict by bringing it out into the open and discussing temptations and dangers of such discussions. Some of the questions to be asked here might be:

To what extent do the same words if applied to different subjects such as social organizations and personalities, retain identical meanings? Is one talking about the same thing if one calls both ambivalences of emotion and clashes of interest in industry by the same name of "conflict"?

What are the dangers involved in thinking by analogy (which seems to be one of the inevitable consequences of interdisciplinary discussions)? Can, for example, the idea of "health" legitimately be applied to social organizations, the ideas of "conciliation" or "mediation" to personalities?

How specific can theories be that are supposed to apply to different subject matters? Are we not forced to remain on a very general level of analysis, if we want to formulate propositions equally applicable to psychological and to sociological problems?

Is the purpose of interdisciplinary discussions mainly that of mutual inspiration, or can such discussions legitimately go further to the formulation of specific hypotheses and theories?

References

Dahrendorf, R. (1959). *Class and Class Conflict in Industrial Society*. Stanford: Stanford University Press.

Newman, F. C. (1961). The process of prescribing "Due Process". *California Legal Review, 49*(215): 227–231.

4 [Editors' note:] See previous chapter.
5 [Editors' note:] Later published as Newman (1961).

Chapter 10

Psychological processes evoked by a major psycho-social transition

Unfinished draft presented to Tavistock Research Workshop – March 1974
by John Bowlby
[Editors: Wellcome Collection Archive, PP/BOW/F.3/90]

This is a contribution to the discussion begun by Parkes's memo of
February 1974:

Elements of the Transition Reaction.[1] It is an attempt to apply to our
problem concepts derived from recent work on information processing,
e.g. by Gregory (1970), Broadbent (1973), Treisman (1974).

Whenever a major change occurs in a person's psycho-social environment he is faced with the task of developing a completely new set of plans
for dealing with his situation. A necessary step in achieving this is to relinquish an out-dated model of his world and the plans based on it and to
develop a new model. We know that this is not easily done and that failure
to complete it can result in psychiatric illness.

Let us consider the problems of effecting such change under five heads –

A. the properties and limitations of the cognitive apparatus
B. the conditions that make it easier or more difficult to relinquish an old
   model and the plans based on it and to replace it with a new model
   and new set of plans
C. the special difficulties encountered when the change involves loss, par-
   tial or complete, of an attachment figure
D. the special difficulties encountered by children
E. the special difficulties encountered by vulnerable individuals.

---

1 [Editors' note:] See Parkes, C. M. (1975). Psycho-social transitions: Comparison between
reactions to loss of a limb and loss of a spouse.

A. Properties and limitations of the cognitive apparatus

Two properties of the cognitive apparatus are of great relevance to our problem –

(a) the conservative nature of internal models
(b) the limited capacity of processing channels, which results in the principal channel often being unavailable to deal with anything but immediate current input.

Gregory (1970) advances the view that, because internal models are built up from past experience, they inevitably reflect the past, not the present, "are essentially conservative" (cf. Marris, 1974) and when faced with change show "inertial drag". Whereas internal models are extraordinarily efficient in helping us deal with a stable environment, they are at their worst when the individual is confronted with major change.

Irrespective of the kind of change a person has to deal with, therefore, changing his model and the plans based on it is going to be slow and difficult. It is made more so by the severe limitations on our capacity for processing information.

Work by Broadbent (1973), Treisman (1974) and others shows that, where two or more messages reach us, we can only deal efficiently with one, even though we can monitor the others adopting simple criteria such as references to ourselves by name or items signifying danger. Near total exclusion of all information other than what is being attended to consciously is thus the rule. Only when time allows is it possible to take a model out of long-term store, to reflect on it and to modify it in greater or lesser degree in the light of new information. We should not be surprised, therefore, if the implications for our models and plans of a major psychosocial transition are dealt with only slowly and piecemeal.

Moreover, because of the conservative nature of models, we must expect that, before undertaking the task of modifying models, every effort will be made, first, to demonstrate that no major environmental change has taken place and, when that fails, to try in every way possible to reverse the change.

If a person is to cope successfully with a major change by developing a new environmental model and new plans it is necessary for him to acquire a great deal of information regarding his new situation. This, Hamburg points out, is exactly what those who proved successful set about doing. Signs that a person is not coping successfully with change are (a) failure to review established models with a view to revising them, and (b) failure to seek necessary new information, Murphey et al. (1963).

B.   Conditions that favour relinquishing old models and replacing them with new

Two of the conditions that facilitate relinquishing and replacing models are –

(a)   opportunity to discuss the position with an informed and congenial friend.
(b)   support and encouragement in tackling the task from a trusted companion (attachment figure).

Although in practice these two conditions may become fused, they are logically distinct and are better considered separately.

Since cognitive models are symbolic constructions, to compare information regarding a changed situation with an existing model, to revise that model or to replace it with a new one, requires systematic analysis of discrepancies etc. In any such situation, therefore, whether it be judged favourable or unfavourable, there are great advantages for a person to have an opportunity to check new facts with a friend, to review possible alternative models and to sketch possible new plans.

Discussion with a companion is thus of advantage from a purely cognitive and logical point of view. From the point of view of feeling the position is similar. A perceived change of environment, if unsought and of any size, is felt as, at best, uncomfortable and a little frightening and, at worst, intensely frightening and painful. To take account of change always requires us to explore the unknown; and this is most easily done when we are given support by an attachment figure. George Brown's finding that an intimate relationship protects a person who has experienced a major psycho-social transition from a clinical depression is in keeping with this position, (Brown et al., 1973).

Seen in this light a person suffers a clinical depression when (a) he experiences a major transition which results in all his existing plans based on his out-dated models being frustrated which itself is depressing enough and (b) he feels hopeless about ever replacing his plans or models with updated ones. In despair at effecting any change he withdraws from making further attempts, though he may spasmodically revert to the out-dated model and the plans based on it.

This may be a good moment to refer to the role of lowered self-esteem in depression. A possible way to look at it is as follows –

(i)   whenever one finds oneself incapable of dealing with a situation one's self-esteem is likely to drop, so that anyone despairing of effecting change in his models and plans will also experience lowered self-esteem.
(ii)   since self-esteem is influenced greatly by the amount of support and encouragement a person is currently receiving from his attachment

figures, there will be a tendency for absence of such support, despair at effecting change and lowered self-esteem to go together.

(iii) since self-esteem is also influenced by the amount of support and encouragement a person received from attachment figures during child-hood, a person who lacked such support in childhood will not only start with lowered self esteem but will, for that reason, expect less in the way of current support and be less able to make use of whatever is available than will someone who received strong support during child-hood. For a person to believe that he is unlovable leads him neither to expect support and help nor to recognize and respond to it when it is offered.

C. *Special difficulties arising when transition involves loss of attachment figure*

When a transition to be coped with involves the loss of a principal attachment figure, as in bereavement, the problem is compounded thrice over. First, the transition is of major dimensions involving the principal components of the person's world model. Secondly, the direction of the change is unfavourable and especially painful. Thirdly, the bereaved is robbed of the very person who, in any other change situation, would have been his main support.

Maddison's finding that mourning progresses best when a person receives help and support from understanding relatives and friends is relevant here. (Maddison, 1968; Maddison & Viola, 1968; Maddison et al., 1969; Maddison & Walker, 1967)

(unfinished)

D. *Special difficulties encountered by children*

(not drafted)

E. *Vulnerable individuals and the conditions that have made them so*

(not drafted)

References

Bowlby, J. (1973). *Attachment and Loss, Vol. II. Separation: Anxiety and Anger.* Har-mondsworth: Penguin.

Broadbent, D. E. (1973). *In Defence of Empirical Psychology.* New York: Methuen.

Brown, G. W., Harris, T. O., & Peto, J. (1973). Life events and psychiatric disorders, Part 2: Nature of causal link. *Psychological Medicine, 3*: 159–176.

Gregory, R. L. (1970). *The Intelligent Eye.* London: Weidenfeld and Nicolson.

Maddison, D. (1968). The relevance of conjugal bereavement to preventive psychiatry. *British Journal of Medical Psychology, 41*: 223–233.

Maddison, D. & Viola, A. (1968). The health of widows in the year following bereavement. *Journal of Psychosomatic Research, 12*: 297–306.

Maddison, D., Viola, A., & Walker, W. L. (1969). Further studies in bereavement. *Australia & New Zealand Psychiatry, 3*: 63–66.

Maddison, D. & Walker, W. L. (1967). Factors affecting the outcome of conjugal bereavement. *British Journal of Psychiatry, 113*: 1057–1067.

Marris, P. (1974). *Loss and Change.* Hove: Routledge & Kegan Paul.

Murphey, E. B., Silber, E., Coelho, G. V., Hamburg, D. A., & Greenberg, I. (1963). Development of autonomy and parent-child interaction in late adolescence. *American Journal of Orthopsychiatry, 33*: 643–652.

Parkes, C. M. (1975). Psycho-social transitions: Comparison between reactions to loss of a limb and loss of a spouse. *The British Journal of Psychiatry, 127*: 204–210.

Treisman, A. M. (1974). Selective attention in man. *British Medical Bulletin, 20*: 12–16.

Appendix

Elements of the Transition Reaction by Colin Murray Parkes, March 1974.

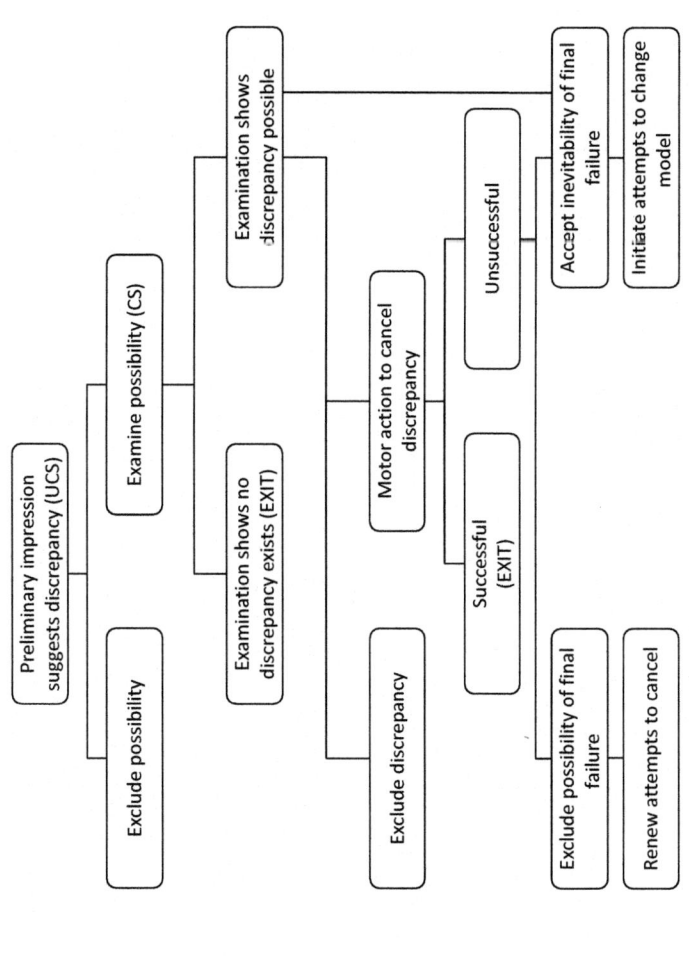

Part 4

Retrospective reflections

Chapter 11

Interview with Alice Smuts

[Editors: Wellcome Collection Archive, PP/BOW/A.5/2]

Interview – June 6, 1977

S:[1] An English paediatrician, Hector Cameron (1918), wrote a book called *The Nervous Child*, published in 1918, that was quite influential in America.

B: Quite influential in this country, too. It was the nearest thing that a paediatrician had come to dealing with these problems. I'd have to read it again to know what its orientation was.

S: You don't remember it having much influence on what you did?

B: No, it had no influence on what I did. Let me tell you what did have an influence on what I did. I went to Cambridge to read medicine, not because I was very enthusiastic about medicine, but because I really didn't know quite what else to do; my father, as you probably know, was a surgeon. And without over-influencing me, he suggested that I read medicine. And once I was at Cambridge reading medicine, I got interested in what we would now call developmental psychology. I was in Cambridge from 1925 through to 1928, and during my third year, having taken the natural sciences tripos my first two years, during my third year I read psychology. And I decided to take it up – whatever that meant!

I proceeded to give up medicine in the summer of 1928, and became interested in what you might call progressive education so I spent the next twelve months in progressive schools. The second two terms, from... [Editors: text missing]... was analytically

---

1 [Editors' note:] Alice Smuts used archival research and interviews to reveal the way inter-related movements—social and scientific—combined to transform the study of the child. She identified social reformers, philanthropists, and progressive scientists including John Bowlby, who established new institutions with new ways of studying children. Smuts, A. (1995, 2008).

oriented.[2] After I'd been there six months and the administrative and financial tangles of the school were still serious, John Alford[3] said to me, "Look – this is no place for you to stay, what you ought to do is to complete your medical training and then train as a child psychiatrist," – I'm not sure he used that phrase, but that's what he meant – "and also train in the psychoanalytic tradition. There are two places in London where you can do a training; one is the Tavistock Clinic and the other is the Institute of Psychoanalysis." Neither of which, I suppose, I'd heard of – well, maybe I had just heard of them. At the time, this was very unpalatable advice; I had no desire to go back and finish my medical training. But fortunately, I took his advice and, in fact, that autumn I started at University College Hospital doing the clinical training. And as regards analytic training, I think he probably said, "Well, the Tavistock group is a bit amateur, I think the psychoanalytic group is more professional; perhaps on balance it might be a better place to train." Anyway, I did in fact sign up with the psychoanalytic group, not the Tavistock. I came into the field, you see, from a residential place for maladjusted children. John Alford saw the present-day problems of these children in terms of their pasts. He first alerted me to all the things which I have thought interesting. He did a Ph.D. in history of art and got a chair at Toronto; he became an American subject in the end. He died ten years ago. He was a very nice man, whom I kept up with very closely; a very gifted person and a great influence on me. That's how I started, you see; it had nothing to do with paediatrics at all.

S: Were there many residential schools for maladjusted children here? Because they were not founded until later in the United States.

B: There were quite a few.

S: They had schools for the mentally retarded, but not for the maladjusted.

B: There were quite a few. For example, there was the American, Homer Lane,[4] who ran a school in this country between 1913 and 1918. It was called the *Little Commonwealth*, and was a very influential venture, especially because it inspired Neill[5] to start *Summerhill*. There have been a fair number of those places, always run by one gifted

---

2 [Editors' note:] This was Priory Gate school in Norfolk.

3 [Editors' note:] John Alford was the headmaster of Priory Gate school.

4 [Editors' note:] Lane, H. (1928) *Talks to Parents and Teachers*, one of the ten books Bowlby cited that had most influenced him. Bowlby, J. (1979) The ten books which have most influenced my thought, 24th October 1979, PP/BOW/A.1/8

5 [Editors' note:] Neill, A. S. (1960). *Summerhill: A Radical Approach to Child Rearing*, foreword by Erich Fromm.

individual who'd collected around himself a few like minded spirits; so long as he lasted things went in a certain direction.

S: In America, when you say progressive education, you immediately think of John Dewey.[6] Same type of influence over here?

B: His influence over here was very much diluted, I presume; one never heard his name over here.

S: The school that you went to – ?

B: I don't think it was consciously influenced by Dewey, no.

S: So when you said, progressive education – you didn't mean that tradition.

B: In this country, there are various traditions in progressive education. If you put the emphasis on progressive, you usually think of A.S. Neill. A.S. Neill was very influential in this country in drawing attention to the limitations of punishment and the need to approach difficult children in a different way. Because, by definition, they were all failures of a disciplinary regime. So you couldn't go on doing it that way – you had to find some other way. A.S. Neill was the most influential figure in this country, for progressive education of that sort apart from Homer Lane, who preceded Neill. Whether they influenced each other, I don't know. But they were both operating in the twenties.

   All the things which I am talking about now stemmed from those two people. They incorporated quite a bit of psychoanalysis, but essentially they started a new, different tradition. Insofar as I've got a distinctive point of view (and in 1936 when I entered child psychiatry I had a distinctive point of view which was neither the current child guidance one nor the psychoanalytic one) I got it from that tradition.

S: Yours is a very different background, I think, from any of the child psychiatrists interviewed by Milton Senn.[7]

B: Well, I've always been very clear in my own mind that that was where all my own ideas started. When I went to Canonbury (London Child Guidance Clinic) as a learner, I brought that point of view plus a psychoanalytic point of view which I'd been imbibing in the preceding five years.

S: And then you said that what you learned there was derived from the psychiatric social workers rather than the psychiatrists.

---

6 [Editors' note:] Dewey, J. (1938). *Experience and Education.*

7 [Editors' note:] Milton Senn was a child psychoanalyst and child psychiatrist who emphasized value of interdisciplinary work, bringing together social workers, early childhood educators and child development specialists. He did a series of interviews with renowned child psychiatrists including John Bowlby. Senn, M. (1977).

B: Yes.

S: What about the educational psychologists? Aside from Lucy Fildes[8] who you said did influence you, did you get much from them?

B: I don't really think I did, to be honest. They were interested in learning difficulties and so on, and I was interested in what we would now call family relationships, personal relationships. And they weren't – so really and truly, I didn't get much from them. I liked them, I respected them, but they were peddling a rather different commodity.

Interview – July 23, 1977

Before the interview actually started Dr. Bowlby and I had been reviewing a conversation he had had with my daughter Barbara concerning the differences between the research tradition and the clinical tradition and the difficulty of working in both worlds. It is this conversation Dr. Bowlby is referring to at the beginning of the interview. – A. Smuts.

B: Now I think that what I was talking about to Barbie was that the mental viewpoints of the clinician and of the research worker are quite different, and they're properly different. I wasn't talking about antagonism between the two, that wasn't in my mind; I was talking about their incompatibility, that the two frames of reference are quite distinct and in certain senses incompatible. Very few people realize that these are two distinct worlds, and that when you are operating in the one world it is proper to have one frame of reference; and when you cross the road and are operating in the other world, it is proper to have a quite different frame of reference.

Now when I formulated that to myself – and I would date it around about 1947 or 1948, soon after the War, but I may be wrong – when I formulated that to myself, it helped me a great deal. When I say "the other side of the road", this is what I mean… The Tavistock Clinic was in Beaumont Street. Then I used to go around the corner from one building to the other, to the research unit there. One took part in a research conference one morning, and in a clinical case conference another morning. Now, the way one thinks and operates in these two conferences is totally different. The average research worker cannot understand the fuzzy-headedness of the clinician, and the clinician cannot understand the remoteness of the research worker. Each finds the other world alien.

---

8 [Editors' note:] Lucy Fildes was a psychologist at the first Child Guidance Clinic set up in 1928.

The reason why so few people do, in fact, combine the two is because they don't realize that you've got to change your frame of reference. When you're operating as a clinician you're concerned with the individual case with all its peculiarities and idiosyncrasies. Your task is to understand the whole problem and do something about it. You draw on what scientific understanding you've got or think you've got; but that never solves a particular clinical problem. You've got to take a lot of leaps in the dark, you've got to use whatever experience you think you've had, and whatever hunches you've got, to work by guess and by God. You've got to take some action, do something. This is also true of the farmer, as a practical man; he's got to solve the problem of making his living on his particular stretch of ground. The agricultural research worker is a completely different animal. The same relationship is true between the engineer and the metallurgist.

Now the scientist is trying to unravel the problems of a particular limited bit of the field, which he has selected partly because he happens to be interested in it, and partly because he thinks he's got some research tools which will enable him to come up with some intelligent answers. But it's always a bit of the field; a small bit. It may be an important bit, or it may be an awfully unimportant bit; anyway it's only a bit. So in one role one is dealing with a messy totality, and in the other with a relatively clean little bit. When you're working as a research worker, you are trying to be precise and rigorous, to get the data tabulated, to scrutinize the data and examine the relationship between data and theory, and theory and data, and all that sort of thing – on a limited front.

When you're a clinician you have no time for that. It's totally inappropriate, it's fiddling. You're dealing with the patient's problems as best you can, and cracking on with it. I've often remarked that in the clinical field you're often applying a theory, which in the research field you're testing to find out if it's true. The point I want to make is that each point of view is appropriate within its own world, and is totally inappropriate in the other world. Unless you realize that, you can't operate in both. To me it's a very simple lesson but it's one that very few people understand... Or perhaps a fair number of people understand it, but not many find it at all congenial to work in both.

S: Can you talk about why you have, and how you have?

B: Well, I don't know. I've had in my personal life representatives of each model. My father was a surgeon, a practicing surgeon. He did a bit of research when he was a young man and he wrote a textbook of surgical pathology which went through many editions, but essentially he was not a researcher. Well then at Cambridge one was exposed to the research tradition, and also after I left Cambridge, when I came to London to read medicine, I'm not sure if I told you this or not, I shared rooms in Camden Town with a young economist.

S: No, you didn't tell me.

B: Well this is very important. Very sadly, he was drowned in 1948 in a holiday accident. Well, Evan Durbin was his name, he was a year older than me, a friend of my brother's at Oxford, actually. He read zoology, and then switched to economics and politics. He came to London the same year as I did, with a junior job first at University College and then at the London School of Economics. He was at the London School of Economics until the War. From 1929 to 1939, we lived in the same house most of the time. Now he was an academic, but he was an academic whose aim in life was to be a politician. In fact, he fought two elections in the 1930s on behalf of the Labour Party; he fought in 1931 and 1935. He won a seat in 1945 and he was a junior minister in the Atlee Labour government from 1946 to 1948.

Well, Evan was – he was a very close personal friend – he was a remarkable fellow, as many people would testify. My family tradition was that you became a clinician and you turned your back on these ivory towers of universities. Evan Durbin represented the other side. Also I should mention that my younger sister married a friend of Evan's, also an economist, who was a fellow of New College (Oxford) at that time; so I was exposed to quite a strong academic influence.

When I was at Cambridge in the twenties, I used to go over to Oxford, and from then on until the War, we used to have long discussions. It was always necessary for me to give good reasons why psychoanalysis "and all that" was about important things. The intellectual climate in which I was living was one where one had to think rigorously and give good reasons and good evidence for one's statement. The notion of being an academic was never in my mind, I don't think it's ever been in my mind. So, I followed, you might say, in my father's footsteps of becoming a specialist, a clinician. But living, as I was, with academics, they were a major influence too.

There are three chapters. First was Evan Durbin. He encouraged me to think of myself as an academic, not to *become* an academic, but to think of myself as having an academic orientation. That's very important, because otherwise I wouldn't have. I remember he encouraged me to register as a PhD student at University College, which I did though I never completed the degree. We wrote a book together before the War, which I don't suppose you have ever heard of...

S: Tell me about it.

B: I'll tell you, it was in about 1936, 1937, when it was evident that War was coming. A British academic, a political scientist – George Catlin – and Evan Durbin got together a symposium. The book was called *War and Democracy.*[9] Well, like many other symposia, it had good contributions and less good. About half the volume was taken up with a contribution, or pair of contributions, by Evan and myself. 150 pages, in fact. And because the reviewers all said this was very interesting and the rest wasn't, our stuff was published separately. It appeared later as *Personal Aggressiveness and War*[10] by Durbin and Bowlby. I can give you a copy. It's a strange book – Evan wrote fifty pages, a fifty page essay, and I wrote a hundred page appendix, which is a little unusual. My appendix reviewed the evidence. The reason I'm referring to that is because it was very typical for Evan to initiate a thing of that sort and, you might say, to drag me in on it. It was my first venture into a quasi-academic sort of article. Anyway, that was the Thirties.

Now, I may have told you that I was very lucky during the War because, when I was drafted into the Army in 1940, it was within the Army psychiatric group which was Tavistock-oriented because the medical director of the Tavistock pre-war, J. R. Rees, was the consultant in psychiatry to the Army. A number of Tavistock people had entered the Army; and a little later a fair number of people like myself who were analysts or analytically oriented, people of that ilk, were recruited into Army psychiatry, too. Well, to cut a long story short, I got mixed up in officer selection very early on; in fact, I did one of the early trials. In 1942 the Officer Selection Boards were introduced and I was on Officer Selection for the next three and a half years. After spending about six months in an operating unit, I was dragged out to join the research and training unit.

I was given the task of validating the selection procedure. Now, my qualifications for this were pretty sketchy, but I was working with three academic psychologists. One of them had a medical degree and was therefore classified as a psychiatrist, but actually he had had a junior job in the Edinburgh Department of Psychology – that was Jock Sutherland.[11] Another was an education psychologist, Ben Morris;[12] and a third was clinical psychologist, Eric Trist.[13] Now we four – two medicals, two non-medicals – were responsible for the technical side of this Research and Training Center from autumn of 1942 until the end of

9 [Editors' note:] Catlin, G. & Durbin, E. F. M. (eds.) (1938). *War and Democracy.*
10 [Editors' note:] Durbin, E. F. M., & Bowlby, J. (1939). *Personal Aggressiveness and War.*
11 [Editors' note:] John ("Jock") Sutherland was Clinical Director of The Tavistock Clinic from 1947-68. Sutherland, J., ed. (1971).
12 [Editors' note:] Ben Morris was an educational psychologist who later became Professor at the Institute of Education, Bristol. Morris, B. (1971).
13 [Editors' note:] Eric Trist developed the organisational concept of socio-technical systems and became chair of the Tavistock Institute of Human Relations. Trist, E., & Bamforth, K. (1951).

the War, 1945. So you see I had three solid years working in what was, not an academic center, but a practically oriented research center. That was invaluable experience for me. It was really a sort of post-graduate training in psychology.

The person to whom I owe most was Eric Trist. He's number two in my list. Evan Durbin is number one, Eric Trist is number two, historically speaking. Eric Trist was a very, very important figure in my life at that time. He's a brilliant person who is his own worst enemy. He's immensely generous to everyone, to all his colleagues, and helps enormously with all their production but tends to neglect his own interests. Anyway, I was one of the people whom he helped. I owe him an enormous amount... what knowledge of psychology I've got, I owe to him. And you see, I was under his influence from 1942. After the war all four of us joined the Tavistock, so we went together straight from one setting to the other.

S: Did you?

B: Oh, that was very important, yes. You see during Army service, a group of psychiatrists and psychoanalysts and clinical psychologists were working together, first of all on officer selection and later on the resettlement of ex-prisoners of war. I wasn't mixed up in that, but Eric Trist was. In addition to the four I've named there were at least another dozen who had worked together in the Army in an operational field but with a research component – it was we who became the post-war Tavistock. I was the only qualified analyst of that group. Though there were other analysts in the Army who were certainly influential, including Adrian Stephen, Virginia Wolff's brother, whom I knew well.

As regards the post-war Tavistock, I haven't mentioned all the relevant names. The four of us I have mentioned were four out of the seven or eight who were influential in developing the post-war Tavistock. As far as I was concerned, I'd been working with these people in the Army and I was working with them again. It was a straight transition, straight out of uniform into civil life – with the explicit intention of doing in civil life the sorts of things we'd been doing in the Army. Well, the notion of developing not only a clinical service but a research side was natural to us, it was the obvious thing to do because that was what we'd been doing in the Army. In officer selection, to take an example: on the one hand we had pioneered a practical technique of selecting officers; on the other hand, we had organized a Research and Training Center which was set up to monitor the techniques and adequacy of the procedures. So we had these two components. I had worked first of all in the field and then back in the research center; so this was a natural way to operate as far as I was concerned.

Consequently, when I joined Tavistock in 1946, my priorities were these: First, we had to have a decent clinical service, because without a decent clinical service, we couldn't train and we couldn't do research, so priority number one: clinical service. Priority number two: training, because, as I said, government policy was to have this type of service right through the country, and there were precious few trained people and very few training programs. So my second concern was to set up this type of training. Noel Hunnybun[14] joined me in 1946, and from Autumn 1946 we were providing a clinical service and a training program. The third thing was to set up research. And I managed to get that started in 1949. I mentioned Evan Durbin as a very crucial figure through the Thirties, Eric Trist as a very crucial figure through the Forties, and from 1954 there was Robert Hinde,[15] the ethologist. He was a crucial figure for me through the Fifties and the early Sixties. Those have been the three, and it is to those three people that I dedicated my second volume.

S: Yes, I noticed Hinde, but the other two names were not familiar to me. I noticed the dedication to Ursula in the first volume. Talking about Hinde kind of leads us into the next thing that I'd really hoped you'd want to talk about, and that is, how you came to be influenced by ethology.

B: Well, you see, I can pick up really in 1948, 1949. I got on to this separation story before the War, and I probably talked to you about that on the other tape.

S: No, you didn't.

B: Didn't I? I've got to go back a bit, I think.

S: Fine.

B: I think I was saying to you that when I came into child guidance work there were two contrasting theoretical outlooks. The social workers were concerned mainly with the current social situation of the child; psychoanalysts were concerned with the child's internal phantasy world. What no one was interested in then, I thought, were the effects of the real experiences that a child has had during his earlier life, which become, as it were, incorporated into his personality and which affect the way he reacts to the current situation. The orientation which I've always plugged has been the immense importance of earlier environment for understanding how a person functions. It's not all just fantasies, its real experience.

14 [Editors' note:] Noel Hunnybun was a psychiatric social worker and influential in the development of Child Guidance Clinics as well his work at the Tavistock Clinic.

15 [Editors' note:] Robert Hinde, renowned ethologist whose research provided new insights into the development of social bonds in primates. Hinde, R. (1970). *Animal Behaviour: A Synthesis of Ethology and Comparative Psychology.*

When I worked at the school, I'd been exposed to that sort of thinking. There was at least one boy there who was, as I would categorize him now, an "affectionless thief". Very dour, remote, an intelligent boy who had been expelled from one of the better known schools for stealing, and who, obviously, was a very light-fingered chap. It was the conventional wisdom of the school to attribute his present condition to his early experiences; he was illegitimate, he'd been brought up for a time by what was allegedly a very rigid nurse and, as I would say now, he'd had no mother figure, really. Anyway, I was alerted to regard that sort of experience as being of consequence. As a result, when I started work at the Child Guidance Clinic, I was interested in that sort of thing.

I remember one particular small boy of about eight who was in constant trouble and seemed impervious to praise or blame. He was very delinquent, and he'd had a disastrous early life. He'd been for nine months in a hospital without any visiting between the age of eighteen months and two years and three months and he had never made any emotional relationship with his parents since. My inclination was to say that his present condition was caused by that experience. And then another child turned up – a little girl – with a very similar condition and a very similar story. So generalizing from a sample of two, I concluded that that causes this. Well, this idea was regarded as mad at the time. But I began collecting other cases.

In addition to doing the book on *Personal Aggressiveness and War*, really to meet Evan Durbin's wishes – I was also working on a monograph, *Forty-four Juvenile Thieves*.[16] It was not published until 1944, but I had got it drafted in 1940. In it I compared forty four children seen at the clinic who stole with forty four other children, also patients at the clinic, who did not steal. And I drew attention to the prevalence of separation experiences, the long separations from family before the age of five, as being a crucial variable. I read a brief paper about it in 1939 [to the British Psychoanalytical Society] which was regarded with considerable scepticism. The full paper was published in the *International Journal of Psycho-Analysis* in 1944, and I got it republished as a monograph in 1946. Now that got around a bit amongst my professional colleagues, including Ronald Hargreaves. He was pre-war Tavistock, exactly my contemporary, and also in the Army where I got to know him. After the War, although he was one of the Tavistock group as we called ourselves, he didn't return to the Tavistock but took the post of Chief of the Mental Health Section of the World Health Organization in Geneva. He was a very able chap.

Now, in 1949 – he'd only been there a year or so – he invited me to do a short term contract with World Health, to write a report on juvenile delinquency. After thinking about it, I decided I didn't particularly want

16 [Editors' note:] Bowlby, J. (1944).

to do juvenile delinquency, so I wrote back and said, "Look, that doesn't suit me too well, but if any else to do with children turns up, I might find it of interest." Well, within a month or two he'd written back and asked, would I undertake a study of the mental health problems of homeless children. And I said yes. I spent about six months of 1950 working from Geneva, on a short-term contract, to prepare a report. In the end I did this monograph for them, *Maternal Care and Mental Health*.[17]

I spent six weeks travelling on the continent collecting material and five weeks in the States. I met a large number of people concerned with child psychiatry and child care problems and I got references to most of the literature. I read the stuff up which I hadn't been able to do before because, what with the Army and developing a department at the Tavistock, I had had no opportunity to catch up with the literature. I wrote the report which came out the following year and which turned out, as you probably know, to be a best-seller.

S: And had world conferences organized and...

B: Yes, it really had an effect. Well, now, I'll tell you the circumstances. I was in the employ of the World Health Organization, and as far as I was concerned it was an opportunity to present the case that early experiences of certain specified sorts have adverse effects. Because that was what no one would believe. People in adult psychiatry regarded it was hooey, people in psychoanalysis regarded it as hooey.

S: Did they?

B: Not all of them, but most of them.

S: Because there had been studies of children in institutions who had been separated from parents...

B: Oh, yes. And those were all grist to my mill. Psychoanalysts, certainly in this country under Ernest Jones and Melanie Klein, held a contrary view. It was almost a dogma that we should not be concerned with real parents, but with the child's conceptions and images and fantasies of parents. And it's not much of an exaggeration to say that in 1939, when I read a paper,[18] the received wisdom in the British Psychoanalytical Society was that real experience is irrelevant, and also that it is almost heretical to pay attention to real experience because if you pay attention to real experience you do not pay attention to the much more important fantasies. And I held very strong views of an opposite sort. Now, I don't want to say that every analyst was hostile to my point of view; that isn't true, but it was a minority position, undoubtedly. I would say it's been a minority position until the very recent years, in Britain. So this was a golden opportunity for me to set the whole thing out, and make my case.

---

17 [Editors' note:] Bowlby, J. (1952).
18 [Editors' note:] Likely Bowlby, J. (1940).

Well, I succeeded in doing so in the sense that it did make people sit up and take notice. I had deliberately selected separation, disruptions of bonds, discontinuities – I had deliberately selected those experiences, not because I thought they were the most important or the most common, but because they were the least controversial; I mean that these events had either occurred or they hadn't, they were well documented, in principle. Whereas, what at the time you could not do, partly because of the climate of opinion and partly because there were no adequate research techniques – you could not examine parental attitudes or the way parents treat children.

Now, a lot of people preach to me about this: "We think that the way parents treat children is much more important than all this business about separation." So I say, "Yes, I thought that forty years ago but I wasn't allowed to say it." At that time, it was regarded as monstrous prejudice to say that a parent was rejecting a child. It's honestly true to say that in some discussions which I've had with psychoanalysts, you might have thought there was no such thing as a battered baby, that parents were either all sweetness and light or else that everything adverse that happened to a child was the result of the child's own difficult behaviour. Anyway, I took another point of view, as you've seen.

Now, that publication, *Maternal Care and Mental Health*, was immensely important for me. It is in two parts. Part one, the evidence that these things are important; part two, what you do about it, practically. What was totally missing – or almost totally missing – from that monograph was any discussion of how it happens – by means of what psychological processes do those experiences have those effects. I remember a review by Winnicott in which he was more than critical that that part of the story had been left out. My answer was that I had written the report in about three months, so how could anyone expect me to have done any more? Anyway, I didn't know, and I didn't think anyone else knew either. So, to cut a long story short, I'd produced this report (it was actually in print in the spring of 1951) but there was a great gap still unfilled. By then I was giving some thought to it.

One could put it in this form now: if the disruption of a bond is important, what is the nature of the bond that's disrupted. I didn't think there was any obvious answer to that one. At that time, the conventional wisdom was that infants are only interested in mothers because mothers feed them. I was profoundly unimpressed by that – I just didn't think it was true, I *knew* it wasn't true. There was a lot of fancy talk about breast-feeding and bottle-feeding and so on; I regarded it all as rubbish. It was completely contrary to my clinical experience; there were very loving mothers who had bottle-fed their babies and some very rejecting mothers whom I met in the clinic, women who were obviously very hostile, who had breast-fed their babies. And it seemed to me the feeding variable was totally irrelevant, or almost totally irrelevant. So I was unimpressed by the conventional wisdom, but I had nothing in particular to put in its place.

It was then, and I can tell you when it was, it was July of 1951, that a young psychologist from the London School of Economics by the name of Norman Hotoph mentioned to me the existence of Lorenz's work on imprinting, about which I'd never heard. So we got hold of his well known paper on the companion in the bird's world published in Germany in 1935,[19] a translation of which had appeared in an American ornithological journal called *Auk*. We got hold of a copy of that from somewhere or other. This was in the days before any photostats or xeroxes or anything, so we got a lot of it typed out because we had only borrowed it from a library. Well, that was the start of my interest in imprinting as: a) a strong bond, b) nothing to do with food, c) something which happens very fast and firmly. This appealed to me, it seemed right.

It happened that that summer we spent our summer holiday up in Scotland, Wester Ross, in the vicinity of my father-in-law, Ursula's father, who was living up there and who was an ornithologist. Among other things, he'd been on expeditions with Julian Huxley, and Julian Huxley and his wife were staying up there with him for a week. I'd met Julian Huxley before, but I saw much more of him on this occasion. I inquired very tentatively, did he know anything about Lorenz or ethology? This led to a very enthusiastic commendation from Huxley who knew him very well and who had done work of his own in the field. Also he had written the Foreword to the English translation of *King Solomon's Ring*[20] which was due out during that winter; he would send me a proof copy when it came, which I duly got in October. That fall I got hold of *King Solomon's Ring* three months before anyone else. Huxley had also given me the name of Tinbergen's book *The Study of Instinct*[21] which had just been published. All this was with Julian Huxley's immense enthusiasm behind it. The more I read of this stuff, the more fascinating I found it. I really spent the whole of 1951–1952 winter mugging up ethology. From that day on, I was completely sold on ethology.

In the spring of 1952 – March 1952 – there was a conference in Oxford convened by the Mental Health Research Fund. About fifty people were invited to attend, mostly psychiatrists, but a certain number of neurophysiologists, neuroanatomists, biochemists as well, to review the state of mental health research in this country. Various people were invited to give papers and others were invited to open discussions. I may have been invited to open a discussion, I can't remember. Anyway, I wasn't invited to give

19 [Editors' note:] Lorenz, K. (1937).
20 [Editors' note:] Lorenz, K. (1952).
21 [Editors' note:] Tinbergen, N. (1952).

a paper. But to cut a long story short, I forwarded a paper about the relevance of ethology to psychiatry which was circulated with the other papers.[22] Well, that was a great success. It was a great success partly because it was completely new and no one had ever heard of ethology before. Everything else was fairly well-known stuff, this was something quite different.

S: A breakthrough, really.

B: Yes, well, it was a trifling little paper, but still it opened a new window. And this is where Ronald Hargreaves comes back into the scene, this Tavistock man who was at the World Health Organization. He was at the conference, and he was greatly taken by two papers, one of which was mine and one of which was a paper on electro-encephalograms by a man called Grey Walter.[23] And he decided that World Health should convene a study group around these areas. I'm not sure how much you know about this, this WHO study group?

S: That's not the one that Macy financed, and then there were the three volumes published on…

B: Four volumes published by Tanner and Inhelder,[24] yes.

S: Yes, I've read those.

B: Well, that's how the World Health one started. Lorenz was there. And Lorenz was there because I had called Ronald Hargreaves' attention to his work the preceding year. Being in Geneva with Lorenz for four consecutive years was very important to me. Not to mention Piaget and various other people. It was Lorenz who told me about Hinde.

S: Was Hinde at Cambridge at that time and you hadn't known he was working in this…?

B: Well, Hinde was a very young man then. He is fifty five now and I'm talking about 1954, so he was then thirty two. Madingley[25] had only just started. Hinde had been in the Air Force during the War – he was in coastal command, piloting anti-submarine flying boats. After the war he went to Cambridge and did a zoology degree, and then to Oxford and did his Ph.D. So in 1954 he'd only just got back to Cambridge – he'd been back there a couple of years, maybe. He and I met in February 1954. Thanks to my having started the ball rolling, what is now the Royal College of

---

22 [Editors' note:] Bowlby, J. (1953a). The contribution of studies of animal behaviour.

23 [Editors' note:] Walter Grey, W. (1953). *The Living Brain.*

24 [Editors' note:] Tanner and Inhelder, (1953-1956) Meetings One to Four of the World Health Organization *Study Group on the Psychobiological Development of the Child,* Geneva, (Tanner & Inhelder, 1953-1956). Members included, John Bowlby, Konrad Lorenz, Margaret Mead, Jean Piaget and Grey Walter, with guests at sessions including Erik Erikson, Von Bertalanffy, and Julian Huxley.

25 [Editors' note:] The Cambridge University Zoological Laboratory.

Psychiatrists (it used to be the Royal Medico-Psychological Association) had planned a scientific meeting on ethology and psychiatry. The two first people they had invited to speak, Lorenz and Tinbergen I think, had been unable to, so Hinde and I came in as substitutes. We each gave a paper, complementary papers, and then, we had lunch together. This was the first time I had met him; and of course I was vastly impressed. From that time onwards, we saw a great deal of each other. It was a two-way process, because I was immensely indebted to him and equally he claims to have been immensely indebted to us at the Tavistock. He used to come up each week to some research seminars that we were holding at the time, and – he was talking about it just the other day – this was a tremendous experience for him, to come in touch with clinicians. So from 1954 onwards insofar as I was drawing on the ethological ideas I was constantly guided and corrected by Robert. From that point onward for a great many years, before I published anything, I asked for his comment.

S: It's interesting that he is now observing children, isn't it?

B: Oh, yes. Well, you see, this is all part of a saga. He was on birds at that time, entirely. Then he spent some months in the States in the spring or early summer of 1957, and we had a talk in July 1957. He said that he'd been to Madison and seen Harry Harlow's[26] work, which was very exciting, and I must visit him. I was due to go to the Center 1957–1958 – September, I was due to go – that's why I can remember the date so well. So before I went to the States, I'd been alerted by Robert that Harry was the man to see. Now, this was very crucial for Hinde because that led him on to work with monkeys; he decided to work with monkeys then and there, largely because of his initial interest in our work, and then...

S: You're talking about Harlow?

B: No, I'm talking about Hinde.

S: Hinde.

B: Harlow's work had had a completely different inspiration. I don't think Harry had ever heard of anything we were doing. His work was, as I understand it, inspired by René Spitz's work.[27] I may have said this before – I think one can't place too much emphasis on the importance of geography. You know, traditions which are immensely important in the States are of no consequence over here; traditions which are immensely important over here are of no consequence in the States. And

---

26 [Editors' note:] Harlow, H. F. (1958). *The Nature of Love.*

27 [Editors' note:] Renee Spitz, renowned for his observation and filming of the effects of maternal and emotional deprivation on infants beginning in the mid-1930s, including producing a seminal film (1952) and book (1965).

it's fair to say as regards maternal deprivation and all that sort of thing, in this country it's associated mostly with my name and in the States it's associated mostly with Spitz's name. And Harlow had been influenced by Spitz, and he was starting his monkey work in 1956–7–8; yes, he'd only been doing it for a year or so in 1957. So when Robert Hinde was out there, it was natural for him both to pick up on the Harlow findings and also pick up on our findings, and to say to himself: "I'm going to work with monkeys, but I'm going to do it differently to Harry." Which of course he did – completely differently. I'm rather proud that I influenced Robert to come into the field – the monkey field, the primate field – and I was also somewhat influential in getting him some research money, because Frank Fremont-Smith – did you ever meet him?

S: No, but I know his name.

B: He was an immensely important figure in our lives in those days – very excited, very enthusiastic, a convener of minds.

S: He seems to have played the same role with Macy that Larry Frank did, perhaps, with the Rockefeller Group. I don't know if this is a fair comparison...

B: Quite likely. You see, the Macy was a small foundation, I don't know what their annual budget was – small by most standards – and he used it very largely for staging such interdisciplinary conferences. The WHO Study Group was inspired by Frank's Macy conferences. Ronald knew about them, he'd been to them – the model was derived straight from the Macy conferences and was chaired by Frank himself. Ronald Hargreaves was insistent that Frank should be the chairman, because he was such a very good chairman. What Frank did as well, in a very quiet way, was to give research support to some of the people he met at the conferences which he convened. I believe he gave quite substantial sums to Lorenz at that time. He gave us some funds at the Tavistock too; I put him on to Robert and he gave him some funds to start the monkey work – I think that's right. I know he gave him some money, and I think that helped him start the monkey work, I couldn't be quite sure. So I assisted Robert to get off the ground with monkeys. I need hardly say that from that point onwards, his work took off. That was the Fifties. Then it was during my stay at the Center in 1957–1958 that I first heard and met Harry, because in April...

S: Harry Harlow?

B: Yes. In April 1958 he was giving a paper to the – I think it's called – the Western branch of the American Psychological Association in Monterey. I made a point of going down there, and the paper he gave was that little paper that he'd already given as President of the American Psychological Association – "The Nature of Love".[28] I think he'd given

28 [Editors' note:] Harlow, H. (1958).

it in the preceding year. I heard him speak and I saw his films, which had a very powerful effect on me. Then I visited him at Madison on my way back to England; I spent two days there in June. That's the story of how I got into ethology.

S: That's quite a story.

B: I may say, at the same time I was also getting Mary Ainsworth interested in ethology.

S: I was going to ask you how this collaboration came about.

B: It started in 1950 because we had got some small research grants; one from this country which enabled us to appoint Jimmy Robertson,[29] one from the European Division of W.H.O and one from a French source, and surprisingly enough. Subsequently, we got grants from the Macy, and later on from Ford. But anyway, when we got this French money, about which there's quite an amusing story, we were able to advertise for two research psychologists; one senior, one less senior. Mary Ainsworth had just come over to London with her husband who was younger than herself and was doing his Ph.D. at University College; so she was on the market and she applied for the job. One of the people at the Tavistock already knew a bit about her, and said she was a good person. She had been in the Canadian Army Psychological Service – that's where he had known about her. Anyway, to cut a long story short, we appointed her to this post; a three-year post. She was working with us at the Tavistock – 1951–1953 – that's how we got to know each other. And then she went off to Uganda. Her husband had got a job at Makerere College in Uganda and they were out there for a year or two, it wasn't very long. Having been working with us for three or four years, she had become very bitten by all this attachment and separation stuff. And, of course, she's gone on with it ever since. When she was in Uganda, she did a study in the homes of the local people the results of which appeared as *Infancy in Uganda*[30] in 1967. I don't know if you've seen that book?

S: No. I know about it, but I haven't read it.

B: No, that's not surprising. The field work was done in 1954–1955, possibly 1956; it didn't appear for ten years. It's a very good book; in fact, a classic. It's a classic for two reasons. First of all, it is the best study of infancy ever done in a non-Western society; and the other is that it's one of the first studies of infancy in Africa. When Mary went to a conference in Africa and met a lot of African psychologists, she discovered she was famous there because she was the only one who had done such a study, which rather amused her. Anyway, she did that study and then she went back to Baltimore and got a job at Johns Hopkins.

29 [Editors' note:] Robertson, J. (1952).
30 [Editors' note:] Ainsworth, M. D. (1967).

Since then, of course, she has gone up the ladder. That's the story with Mary Ainsworth. And the point is this: we'd become pretty close while she was over here, and we kept up communication, correspondence, when she was in Africa. I wrote to her about ethology. Well, she must have known a bit about it before she went out because I was becoming enthusiastic about it in 1951 and 1952 when she was here; she must have shown a lot of interest in it. But many of the more basic ideas I only grasped subsequently. And I remember having quite prolonged debates on paper about certain things, because various points which I was advancing, which were fairly conventional ethological ones, were totally alien to her and needed a lot of explanation. That's how she became an enthusiastic ethologist, or ethologically oriented person.

S: How many psychiatrists today are knowledgeable, or at least accepting – sorry, they're two different questions. How many are knowledgeable about...

B: Well, knowledgeable – extremely few, I would think. Apart from a few colleagues I would really have difficulty in naming any that I thought were reasonably knowledgeable. I'm sure there must be some, but they're pretty scarce. One of course, in the States, one which you know well, is Dave Hamburg. But. no, the answer is jolly few, very few.

S: Has William Kessen ever corresponded with you on this? He seemed to say a few things in...

B: Yes, but Kessen's a psychologist; you asked me about psychiatrists.

S: That's right.

B: If I stick to psychiatrists, the answer is jolly few. I really do have difficulty in thinking who they would be. But the number who think it's interesting and reputable is now fairly large. It is now accepted, but it's still a mystery-land, I would think, to most of them. Insofar as reputable people like Robert Hinde, who is now a Fellow of the Royal Society, is working in this field, and other people like myself think it's valuable – they say, "It must be all right but we don't really quite see how it fits in, it doesn't seem to have paid off very much yet anyway." This is my impression. The notion that it's all baloney is certainly no longer in fashion.

S: Not even among anthropologists any more.

B: Is that so?

S: Well, they're changing.

B: People are changing, but they change slowly. But I would say that there are very few psychiatrists who understand what ethology has to teach psychiatry, very few. There's a very nice man – a Scotsman – out in Canberra – Scott Henderson,[31] I would count him as one, he does understand what ethology is about.

---

31 [Editors' note:] Henderson S. (1974).

S: Is he the one who did the article on care eliciting behavior?

B: Yes.

S: I read that.

B: You see he knows what it's about. There must be half a dozen others, but it's very small, is my impression. Among psychologists, I'm sure there are many more. There are probably quite a number of psychologists who know about ethology. Even so, many people know about it but haven't understood it.

S: We were talking about Blurton-Jones...

B: Nick Blurton-Jones, he's an ethologist, he's not a psychologist. He's an ethologist. For his Ph.D. he was doing birds. And he came in to study children with Jim Tanner, more than ten years ago now. I don't think he's a brilliantly original mind; I think he's a very capable workman and he's a very good influence. He edited a very useful collection of papers on *Ethological Studies of Child Behaviour* in 1972;[32] but I don't suppose it's been read by more than a handful of psychiatrists. But times change. For instance, Robert was invited to give the Emanuel Miller lecture to the Association of Child Psychologists and Psychiatrists a couple of years ago.[33] And he has published a lot of his monkey stuff in the Journal of Child Psychology and Psychiatry. So again, I suppose, people in child psychiatry are tolerably familiar with ethology and regard it as interesting and perhaps very important, even if they don't know a lot about it. People in adult psychiatry, I suspect, are very hazy about it.

S: That's an interesting point; I hadn't realized that.

B: I would guess that.

S: There were a couple of meetings of the Society – well, this is psychology again, not psychiatry – but meetings at the Society for Research in Child Development on this subject. You had to keep analysts separate from psychiatrists in the 1920s and 1930s.

B: And in this country still today.

S: And today too.

B: Oh, yes. And psychologists distinct from either. No, these are quite distinct traditions.

S: Of course, I know that.

B: Totally different. The relevance of ethology to psychiatry is now recognized as legitimate, possibly interesting. But a sceptical "What's the payoff anyway?" is, I would think, a common attitude.

S: I wondered if you wanted to put something on the tape on some of the points you made in your Maudsley lecture, because this is for an American audience, and I don't know how many of them would be familiar with that

32 [Editors' note:] Blurton Jones, N. (1972).
33 [Editors' note:] Hinde, R. (1976).

paper. I was thinking particularly of these points; it seemed to me very significant. They're in your books, too, but I thought of it as another way of reaching young American students who might not yet have read your books.

B: I'm not averse to doing it at all. *Maternal Care & Mental Health* in WHO format came out in 1951. I may say it was always difficult to get hold of because it was handled in this country by the government stationers (H.M. S.O.), and in the States by Colombia University Press – and neither kept any stock of it. So, in fact, it was very poorly circulated. But the abridged paperback version[34] got more publicity. Marjorie Fry was one of our great women between the War years. She died at the age of eighty-something or other in 1958. She was one of the Fry family, a sister of Roger Fry, the painter. Although she'd never been to University herself, she was invited to become head of one of the Oxford colleges, and later was on the University Grants Committee – she became a great power in the land. She was also a juvenile court magistrate – very charming, very amusing, very intelligent. I got to know her a bit at the outbreak of War, because she came down to live in Cambridge and the London Child Guidance Clinic also emigrated to Cambridge and we ran into each other. She became very interested in the *Forty-four Juvenile Thieves* study of mine, being a juvenile court magistrate. And when *Maternal Care and Mental Health* came out, I no doubt sent her a copy, and she became very enthusiastic. She rang me up and said, "This ought to be more available to the public and in a simpler form: publish it as a paperback." So I said yes – would you like to do it? So, very modestly she said, Well, she'd have a try, she didn't know if she could really manage. She'd send me some samples of her abridgement. Well I didn't think much more of it. About a week later, the sample arrived, and it was admirable. So she did the abridgement and I made some minor revisions and it came out in Penguin. It had to have a new title. I didn't give Penguin the American rights because I wanted it published in the States, on the grounds that Penguin had a very poor circulation in the States – never has had, still don't. And Nina Ridenour, do you know the name?

S: Yes, yes.

B: Well, she became an enthusiast too, and she said she would take the Marjorie Fry abridgement and put it into American, because there were various places where the lingo was not right for America. She did that, and it was going to be published by one of the American publishers.

S: It *was* going to be published?

B: It was *going to be*, but it wasn't. The publishing house, I forget now which one it was, went cold on it. And they didn't do it. Subsequently, I let the Penguin people have the American copyright, but it has never

34 [Editors' notes:] Bowlby, J. (1953b). *Child Care and the Growth of Love.*

sold more than the odd thousand or so copies in the States. I guess the total sales in the States might be 20,000 copies compared to half a million in the rest of the world. And there has been the sales story – a) an English author, b) an English publisher – so very little circulation for the States.

S: I read somewhere about the Washington school in America, being very sympathetic to your work. How did that come about? Well, which school do they mean. Is that the University of Washington or...?

B: No, I think they mean the Washington psychoanalytic group. Now the Washington psychoanalytic group has always been a bit aberrant. You might say the New York Society has been a sort of Mecca – where you learn the truth, the whole truth, and nothing but the truth belongs in New York. Chicago has had its liberal tendencies, with Franz Alexander. Washington has always been much more open-minded and liberal, much more socially oriented. Harry Stack Sullivan was in Washington. He was a powerful influence over there – less so over here. The Washington school of psychoanalysis has always been more oriented towards the kinds of things I'm interested in. But it's always regarded as off-center of the American Psychoanalytic Association. New York Society is in the middle and the other various ones on the periphery. And Washington is on the periphery.[35]

[John Bowlby additions:]
There are three topics which we talked about which have disappeared from the transcripts owing to a breakdown of the tape-recorder. These additions are dated September 1979.
One concerned family therapy.
From the time I first went to the London Child Guidance Clinic and worked with Molly Lowden and Nance Fairbairn I realized that parents' own emotional problems play a large part in the problems presented by their children. I have given some historical examples in a recent paper (*Psychoanalysis as Art and Science*).[36] So I regarded the treatment of parents' problems as just as important as treating the children's. At that time, although I always saw parents during assessment interviews, it was customary for therapeutic work with them to be done by the psychiatric social workers. Fathers, however, tended to be left out altogether unless a crisis arose.
When Noel Hunnybun joined me at the Tavistock in 1946 we began by following the same pattern as before the war. Very soon, however, thanks to a remark by a visiting American psychiatric social worker, we made

---

35 [Editors' note:] Text is cut at this point, as the remainder is mostly Smuts talking at Bowlby.
36 [Editors' note:] Bowlby, J. (1979).

a point of including fathers at the initial interviews and working with them. Some of the psychiatric social workers were very skilled at working with parents along analytic lines and I did all I could to encourage students to go as far as they could in dealing with parents' emotional problems.

Throughout 1947, however, no one dreamt of seeing more than one member of a family together.

My first family interview took place early in 1948. I had been having regular weekly interviews with an intelligent boy of fourteen or fifteen. He was thoroughly up against his parents and was doing badly at school. In general he was morose and uncommunicative. For reasons I can't remember neither of his parents were being seen by a social worker but, because there was obviously much friction at home, I arranged to see both parents one Saturday morning. When I went to the waiting room and saw all three there together I made the sudden decision to invite them together to my room, without having any plan how I was going to proceed. Discussion soon became lively, however, and mother's constant nagging of her son became very evident. When I asked her what sort of childhood she herself had had she broke down into tears and for the next three quarters of an hour described a long series of distressing events. Her husband had previously known little of this and her son nothing. After about 100 minutes the session ended with each member of the family more insightful and understanding of the other's problems than before. Thereafter I continued to see the boy on his own. But from that day onwards I was convinced of the value of joint family interviews and made a practice of having at least one such during the assessment phase of every case I saw.

It happened that in the summer of 1948 the World Federation of Mental Health held an international conference in London, the first such event after the war. Amongst many other activities, visits were arranged to clinics and hospitals. When the Tavistock entertained visitors, members of staff gave a series of brief papers on the theme of Group Tensions and means of handling them. For example, one paper was about group tensions in industry. To make up the programme I agreed to give an extempore talk about Group Tensions in the Family and I drew for my example on the successful family interview I had had during the previous winter. Subsequently my talk, with others, was prepared for publication in a symposium for a number of the Journal of Social Issues for 1949.[37]

For the next ten years I strove to convince my colleagues in the Department for Children and Parents of the value of joint family interviews but met with considerable opposition, especially from members of staff with a Kleinian orientation. One of them, I recall, accused me of cruelty to the children involved. The only member of staff actively to support me was

---

37 [Editors' note:] Bowlby, J. (1949). This is now the *Journal of Human Relations.*

Molly Mackenzie, a child psychiatrist and psychoanalyst. But not until 1960 did things begin to change. That year a Canadian psychiatrist, Freda MacQueen (subsequently Martin),[38] joined us as a registrar. She quickly adopted a joint interview technique and as she progressed to senior registrar and staff status had a powerful influence on several members of staff. Although I gave her every encouragement and what help I could, as did Molly Mackenzie, I had too much else on my plate to make any further contribution myself.

An episode that took place in 1952 or 1953 may be of interest. A child psychiatrist, newly promoted consultant, asked me what area of child psychiatry he should adopt as his special field of interest. I offered him two. One was the application of ethological ideas to our work; the other was joint family interviews. Both I believed had great potential but I could not envisage developing either of them myself. What research time I had, I said, would be taken up with separation. To my regret the young consultant did not take up either of my ideas. In the event, I developed the ethological side myself and it was left to Freda Martin – and of course many others elsewhere – to develop family therapy.

The second topic omitted from the tapes was my view on the relation of child psychiatry to pediatrics.

From the time I started clinical work as a medical student my aim was to become qualified as a psychoanalyst and child psychiatrist as soon as I possibly could. Since one of the requirements for being given a Commonwealth Fellowship in child psychiatry was some experience of adult psychiatry, I went straight to the Maudsley the day after I qualified in medicine. The notion of doing paediatrics never occurred to me. Moreover, I set my face against spending any time working for an M.R.C.P., which Aubrey Lewis had strongly advised, and even avoided doing the D.P.M. which was at that time the only psychiatric qualification. Thus I cut all the corners and never did any paediatrics, apart from a rather perfunctory month or two as a medical student. Rightly or wrongly this lack never bothered me particularly. When taxed with having done no general medicine after qualification my retort always was that I would do some more general medicine as soon as my critic had done as much psychology and psychiatry as I had already done physiology and medicine as a medical student.

My position was that analytically oriented child and family psychiatry was as much a discipline of its own as either adult psychiatry or paediatrics were, and that child psychiatry would not progress so long as it was regarded as a sub-specialty of something else and so long as trainees spent some of their best years studying other specialties before coming into child psychiatry. I often used the analogy of the Royal Air Force. Certainly, the Air arm

38 [Editors' note:] Martin, F., & Knight, J. (1962).

had to co-operate with the Army and Navy but it could never do so properly so long as it was a subordinate arm of one of the others. Had it not been that the RAF was set up as a separate service equal to the Army and the Navy we should never have won the Battle of Britain in 1940.

A third topic (which was only touched upon in the interviews) was my relation to the British Psychoanalytic Society. I qualified in 1937 at the age of thirty (much younger than most) and went straight on to train in child analysis. Mrs. Klein was my supervisor. The first case I was allocated was an extremely anxious overactive three-year-old boy whose working-class mother was agitated and depressed. Not only was it the practice for a child analyst never to see parents but Mrs. Klein was profoundly uninterested in any comments I may have made about this poor woman. Nothing about the boy's father or the rest of the family ever reached me. After three months mother was admitted to a mental hospital and the boy's treatment ended. This was regarded by my supervisor as merely an unfortunate interruption of my training and a new case was sought. The second child allotted me was a little girl of two and a half who still wet herself by day and night, and was jealous of the new baby. Once again no interest was shown in mother, let alone father; but mother on occasion insisted on having her say. She also was a troubled woman, and one of the things she told me was that, when pregnant with the child I was seeing, she had attempted an abortion. After a few months the war intervened. When it was over and I was free to resume my training I could not face doing so, however: the absurdity of treating young children and neglecting their parents was too much for me.

Nevertheless, from the time I qualified as an analyst in 1937 I was eager to play an active part in the Psychoanalytic Society. I took some part in scientific meetings, and in the summer of 1939 read a paper on "The Influence of Early Environment on the Development of Neurosis and Neurotic Character"[39] in which I outlined my views, including the adverse effects of prolonged separation, with clinical illustrations drawn from my child guidance experience. Melitta Schmideberg, Melanie Klein's daughter, with whom I was friendly and who agreed with my viewpoint, warned me in advance that neither the topic nor the thesis would be popular. Despite that, however, and despite the fact that I had not followed the tradition of a membership paper by giving a detailed account of the analysis of a patient, I was duly elected a full member. For the first two years of the war activities of the Society were suspended. Ernest Jones took up residence at his country home in West Sussex and, although he came up especially to chair a series of special meetings held during the winter of 1942–43, he never subsequently lived in London; and he took no further part in the Society's affairs.

39 [Editors' note:] Bowlby, J. (1940).

Since the arrival of members of the Viennese Society in 1938 the friction between Melanie Klein's group and Anna Freud's, which had begun in the mid-twenties, threatened the unity of the British Society. Early in 1943 I was posted to Hampstead and thereafter took an active part in trying to ensure that the Society adopted a more democratic constitution and also that it remained unified. In these efforts I supported Adrian Stephen in bringing in a rule to prevent an officer remaining in the same office for more than three years; and subsequently accepted Sylvia Payne's request that I stand for Training Secretary. From 1944 to 1947 I acted in that capacity under her presidency and played a part in planning the two parallel training courses sponsored by the Society. Had I then gone into full time or even half time analytic practice I could almost certainly have become a training analyst, but I had no desire to do so.

Throughout the fifties I continued to play an active part in the Society and presented scientific papers on at least four occasions. One was in connection with the film *A Two-Year-Old Goes to Hospital*;[40] another when I outlined the relevance of ethological ideas to psychoanalysis; the third in summer 1957 when I gave *The Nature of the Child's Tie to His Mother*,[41] which met with an avalanche of criticism, especially from the Kleinians; and the fourth in Autumn 1958 after my return from nine months at the Behavioral Sciences Center, when I presented, *Separation Anxiety*.[42] This gave rise to a very lively and for the most part critical discussion which was continued for a further two meetings. Once again the Kleinians made an organized attack on my position.

During this period, 1956–57 and again 1958–61, I was asked by Sylvia Payne to assist in the administration of the Society and Institute by becoming Deputy President under Donald Winnicott. In this role I chaired the Council. Although in the natural course of things I might well have been elected the next president it had become clear that there would be too much opposition and, with my agreement, those supporting me did not propose me. By then it was evident that I had failed to convince more than a minority of members that my ideas were of value to psychoanalysis and that, even were I to be elected president, it would be an unhappy and unproductive arrangement. Thenceforward my relations with the Society became less close. Though I remained on cordial terms with members and took part in any activities or gave papers to groups whenever invited, I ceased to attend regularly at scientific meetings.

Over the past dozen years a number of Psychoanalytic Societies overseas have invited me to speak and I have always made a point of accepting

40 [Editors' note:] See Robertson, J. (1952).
41 [Editors' note:] Bowlby, J. (1958).
42 [Editors' note:] Bowlby, J. (1960).

whenever possible. Examples are the Italian Society, the San Francisco Society, the Society of Southern California, the Australian Society and the Canadian Society who in 1978 invited me to give their Academic Lecture. On almost all these occasions my remarks have been greeted with interest and sometimes with enthusiasm. This was also the case when I took a minor part in a session on the family at the International Psychoanalytic Congress which was held in London in 1975. On this occasion I had not been invited to be one of the panel of speakers or discussants but during the discussion itself I was invited to join the platform party – a good illustration of my ambiguous relationship with the psychoanalytic movement.

One further point concerns publications. I was keen for my work on *Attachment and Loss* to be published first in a series of papers in the *International Journal of Psychoanalysis* and later as a volume in the *International Library of Psychoanalysis.* Since the editor both of the Journal and of the Library from 1958 to 1968 was my friend, Jock Sutherland, who always took my work seriously, there was no difficulty about this. He was glad to publish the early papers and had also accepted, the first volume for the Library before giving up the editorship. Subsequent editors have also been glad to have the second and third volumes. Throughout these years my concern has been to work with analysts towards a reformulation of psychoanalytic theory and to avoid spending time and energy merely criticizing traditional theory. Though it has been an uphill job I believe the strategy is slowly paying off.

References

Ainsworth, M. D. (1967). *Infancy in Uganda: Infant Care and the Growth of Love.* Baltimore: The Johns Hopkins Press.

Blurton Jones, N. G. (Ed.). (1972). *Ethological Studies of Child Behaviour.* London: Cambridge University Press.

Bowlby, J. (1940). The influence of early environment in the development of neurosis and neurotic character. *The International Journal of Psycho-Analysis, 21*: 154–178.

Bowlby, J. (1944). Forty-four juvenile thieves: Their characters and home-life. *The International Journal of Psychoanalysis, 25*: 19–53.

Bowlby, J. (1949). The study and reduction of group tensions in the family. *Human Relations, 2*: 123–128.

Bowlby, J. (1952). *Maternal Care and Mental Health: A report prepared on behalf of the World Health Organisation as a contribution to the United Nations programme for the welfare of homeless children* (2nd ed.). Geneva: World Health Organization.

Bowlby, J. (1953a). The contribution of studies of animal behaviour. In: J. M. Tanner (Ed.), *Prospects in Psychiatric Research* (pp. 80–108). Oxford: Blackwell.

Bowlby, J. (1953b). *Child Care and the Growth of Love.* Harmondsworth: Pelican.

Bowlby, J. (1958). The nature of the child's tie to his mother. *The International Journal of Psycho-Analysis, 39*: 350–373.

Bowlby, J. (1960). Separation anxiety. *The International Journal of Psycho-Analysis, 41*: 89–113.

Bowlby, J. (1979). Psychoanalysis as art and science. *International Review of Psycho-Analysis, 6*: 3–14.

Cameron, H. (1918). *The Nervous Child*. London: Oxford University Press.

Catlin, G., & Durbin, E. F. M. (Eds.). (1938). *War and Democracy*. London: Kegan Paul.

Dewey, J. (1938). *Experience and Education*. New York: Kappa Delta Pi.

Durbin, E. F. M. & Bowlby, J. (1939). *Personal Aggressiveness and War*. London: Kegan Paul, Trench, Trubner.

Harlow, H. (1958). The nature of love. *American Psychologist, 13*: 573–685.

Henderson, S. (1974). Care-eliciting behavior in man. *Nervous Mental Disorders, 159*: 172–181.

Hinde, R. A. (1970). *Animal Behaviour: A Synthesis of Ethology and Comparative Psychology*. New York: McGraw Hill.

Hinde, R. A. (1976). On describing relationships. *Journal of Child Psychology and Psychiatry, 17*: 1–19.

Lane, H. (1928). *Talks to Parents and Teachers*. London: George Allen & Unwin.

Lorenz, K. (1937). The companion in the bird's world. *The Auk, 54*: 245–273.

Lorenz, K. (1952). *King Solomon's Ring*. London: Methuen.

Martin, F. & Knight, J. (1962). Joint interviews as part of intake procedure in a Child Psychiatric Clinic. *Journal of Child Psychology and Psychiatry, 3*: 17–26.

Morris, B. (1971). An educational perspective on mental health. In: J. D. Sutherland (Ed.), *Towards Community Mental Health* (pp. 31–46). London: Tavistock.

Neill, A. S. (1960). *Summerhill: A Radical Approach to Child Rearing*. New York: Hart Publishing Company.

Robertson, J. (1952). *A Two Year Old Goes to Hospital*. Film. Young Children in Brief Separation Research Project, Tavistock Clinic, London.

Senn, M. J. B. (1977). *Interview with Dr John Bowlby in London, England, 19th October, 1977*. Unpublished. National Library of Medicine, Bethesda, Maryland, USA.

Smuts, A. (1995). *Science Discovers the Child, 1893–1935*. Ph.D. dissertation. University of Michigan.

Smuts, A. (2008). *Science in the Service of Children, 1893–1935*. New Haven, CT: Yale University Press.

Spitz, R. A. (1952). *Psychogenic Diseases in Infancy: An attempt at their classification* [Film]. New York University Film Library.

Spitz, R. A. (1965). *The First Year of Life. A Psychoanalytic Study of Normal and Deviant Development of Object Relations*. New York: International Universities Press.

Sutherland, J. (Ed.). (1971). *Towards Community Mental Health*. London: Tavistock.

Tanner, J. M., & Inhelder, B. (Eds.). (1953–1956). *Discussions On Child Development (4 Volumes)*. London: Tavistock Press.

Tinbergen, N. (1952). *The Study of Instinct*. Oxford: Clarendon Press.

Trist, E. & Bamforth, K. (1951). Some social and psychological consequences of the longwall method of coal getting. *Human Relations, 4*: 3–38.

Walter Grey, W. (1953). *The Living Brain*. London: Duckworth.

Chapter 12

The role of the psychotherapist's personal resources in the treatment situation

31st May 1985 [Wellcome Collection Archive, PP/BOW/K.10/65. Also circulated to the *Bulletin of the British Psychoanalytic Society, 27*(11): 26–30 in 1991.][1]

Since I have never regarded psychotherapy as my principal role in the psychoanalytic world, my aim here is to describe what I have been trying to do and why. Only at the end do I refer to myself as a therapist.

After reading natural sciences and psychology at Cambridge, I worked for a year in a school for maladjusted children in which it was held that the children's present troubles were the result of adverse experiences they had had in their families earlier in life. Working temporarily at the school was a gifted man, John Alford, who had had difficulties of his own and who had had analytically oriented psychotherapy from an American lay therapist then working in England. Alford's advice to me was to complete my medical studies and train at one of the two analytically oriented clinics in London, either the Tavistock, which was eclectic, or else the Psychoanalytic Institute. I opted for the latter and came to London in the Autumn of 1929, aged twenty two, to enter University College Hospital Medical School and to start an analysis with Mrs. Riviere, a non-medical and close friend of Melanie Klein. My aim was to become a child psychiatrist, a specialism just becoming recognized in Britain at that time.

Immediately on qualifying medically in the Spring of 1933, I started working at the Maudsley under Aubrey Lewis to learn adult psychiatry; I also took a patient under supervision at the psychoanalytic clinic and began attending lectures and seminars. This regime continued for the next three years though I did less at the Maudsley and saw more patients for psychotherapy at other clinics. In 1936, I began working part-time at the London Child Guidance Clinic and continued there until 1940, when I became an army psychiatrist.

---

1 [Editors' note:] Published with the permission of the Editor of *Bulletin of the British Psychoanalytic Society.*

Although I had read Freud's *Introductory Lectures* at Cambridge, it was not until I got to London that I read psychoanalysis seriously (always confined to English translations). Though I found the subject matter fascinating and adopted the overall viewpoint, I was dissatisfied with much of the theory. However, I made a point of suspending judgment pending much more experience. As a somewhat arrogant young man with a number of academic friends, mainly in the economic and social sciences, I was in no mood to accept dogmatic teaching. Moreover, my academic friends, although actively interested in psychoanalysis, never ceased to put challenging questions to me; whilst Aubrey Lewis, a keen intellect and sceptic, was always demanding more evidence, as indeed I was myself. My analyst was not altogether happy with my critical attitude and complained on one occasion that I would take nothing on trust and was trying to think everything out from scratch, which I was certainly committed to doing.

My therapeutic work tended to be fairly Kleinian which meant that I gave a great deal of attention to the transference, but ignored the patient's real life experiences, both those of childhood and also later ones. My first supervisor, a Kleinian, was rather a prim old maid and we seemed never to be on the same wave-length. (Later she resigned from the Society). My second was Ella Sharpe, a warm-hearted middle-aged woman who had a good understanding of human nature and a sense of humour. Both had been school teachers before becoming analysts. I suspect I learned a good deal from Ella Sharpe about treating patients as human beings, but it was only later, I believe, that I began helping the patient: this was when I started applying what I was learning in the Child Guidance Clinic about the kind of family experiences that contribute to emotional problems. The patient, a girl in her early twenties, given to hysterical outbursts and depressive symptoms, had always been extremely silent. She was the second in a large family, the eldest also a girl, and the next two younger both boys. Something led me to remark "It sounds to me as though your mother never really wanted you." At that she burst into tears and we began dealing with her difficult family situation in which she had been the unwanted second girl, soon followed by two boys towards whom her mother had always shown extreme favouritism. My first patient, a woman in her late thirties in an acutely anxious and agitated state, was, I can now see, in a condition of seriously disturbed mourning following the death of her mother with whom she had had a pathogenic relationship. Neither I nor my supervisor were in any way aware of that, however, and I'm afraid I helped that patient very little.

By the summer of 1937 I had been in analysis over seven years, and seeing patients under supervision for four, and was becoming restive for qualification. Although Mrs. Riviere was still not satisfied with my progress, she finally agreed, and that summer I became an associate member. Since this does not carry voting rights in the Society, I was eager to take the next step which required reading a paper at a scientific meeting. I also decided to train as a child analyst.

During the years 1936–39 I was slowly waking up to the fact that my ideas were developing in a direction very different from those that were the accepted truths in the British Psychoanalytical Society. At that time, under the influence of Ernest Jones and Melanie Klein, it was held that an analyst should concern himself only with the patient's internal world and that to give attention to his real life experiences could only divert attention from what really matters. My experiences in the child guidance clinic, however, were leading me to an opposite conclusion, namely that one can only understand a person's internal world, and thus see his current situation through his own spectacles, if one can see how his internal world has come to be constructed from the real-life events and situations to which he has been exposed. Furthermore, it was obvious that emotional disturbance and personality disorders could only be prevented from developing if we knew a great deal more about the nature of pathogenic experiences and how they affect psychological development. The upshot was that by 1938–39 I had decided to make a systematic study of the family situations that give rise to psychopathology.

At the child guidance clinic I had seen a number of children referred on account of persistent stealing and truancy, and all of whose personal relationships seemed superficial and shallow. With only one or two exceptions they had a history of grossly disrupted relationships with family during their first five years and it seemed to me probable that their present psychological state was a result of those disruptions. Since this seemed to be a novel idea, I decided to make this a focus of the paper I was to read to the Psychoanalytical Society; and I also decided to collect a series of child and adolescent cases in which stealing was a problem and to compare them with a similar number of other clinic cases in which stealing was not a problem in order to test the idea that persistent stealing and gross disruptions go together.

Meanwhile, during my training in child analysis, my attention was being drawn most forcibly to the way some analysts neglect a child's family. It had been arranged that the supervisor of my first child patient should be Mrs. Klein. The case allotted me was an anxious, aggressive and hyperactive small boy aged three. He was brought to the clinic by his mother whose role was to sit in the waiting room whilst I treated her son. The fact that she was an intensely anxious distressed woman was not regarded as relevant, and I was instructed not to spend time with her, an arrangement I found difficult to bear. After three months word reached me that this woman had been admitted to a mental hospital, which hardly surprised me. When I reported this to Melanie Klein, however, her only concern seemed to be that, since it was no longer possible to continue the boy's analysis, another patient must be found for me. The probability that the boy's behaviour was a reaction to the way his mother treated him seemed altogether to escape her. A comparable, though less dramatic, difference in our outlooks was evident when I began treating the next child.

This experience was a powerful stimulant to me to pursue my chosen field, and at a scientific meeting of the Society in June 1939 I read my paper entitled "The Role of Early Environment in the Development of Neurosis and Neurotic Character" (Bowlby, 1940). Beforehand I had been warned by Mrs. Klein's daughter, Melitta Schmideberg, who was a friend and well disposed to my thesis, that it would meet with much criticism. In the event, however, this was not so. Such criticism as there was, was matched by sympathetic interest, especially from Susan Isaacs, an academic psychologist who supported Mrs. Klein, though also maintaining her broader interests. A month or so later I was duly elected a full member of the Society, though not without some opposition.

This brief paper was published in the *International Journal of Psycho-Analysis* the following year and, apart from an even briefer paper, entitled "Primary Affect Hunger", by David Levy which had appeared in the *American Journal of Psychiatry* in 1937 (but was then unknown to me), was among the first to draw attention to the ill-effects of maternal deprivation (Levy, 1937). During the Autumn and Winter of 1939 I completed a draft of my more systematic study, entitled "Forty-four Juvenile Thieves: Their Characters and Home Life" (Bowlby, 1944); this I submitted to the *British Journal of Medical Psychology*, the editor of which was John Rickman, a relatively senior analyst. He replied fairly favourably but judged that, before publication, it required a discussion of theory.

Meanwhile, the war had broken out. Many analysts left London and others were mobilized into the Emergency Medical Service. One result was that my training in child analysis was interrupted, which had the advantage of avoiding an open clash with my supervisor. I did not resume it after the war. In September 1940 I began five years as an army psychiatrist, all of it spent in Britain and most of it dealing with problems of officer selection. This work, initiated by army psychiatrists, led me to be associated with a number of professional psychologists and resulted in my receiving a training in psychological research. It also led to my becoming one of the group which later became responsible for reorganizing the Tavistock Clinic after the war. Several of its members became close friends. One of these was Jock Sutherland who had had analysis with Ronald Fairbairn in Edinburgh before the war and subsequently did a training in London. Another was Eric Trist, a clinical and social psychologist, who acted as my research supervisor in the army and as a consultant to my research group for ten years or more at the Tavistock after it.[2]

At the beginning of 1943 the Research and Training Centre for Officer Selection had moved to Hampstead, and this gave me the opportunity to

2 [Editors' notes] For information about those mentioned here, readers are referred to Dicks, H. V. (1970) *Fifty Years of the Tavistock Clinic*.

participate in meetings of the British Psychoanalytical Society, which was then undergoing convulsions as a result of the conflict between Melanie Klein's group and the group from Vienna headed by Anna Freud. Although my training had been Kleinian, I quickly identified myself with a number of other indigenous British members, of whom Sylvia Payne and Adrian Stephen were leaders, who were concerned to hold both groups within the Society and to avoid the threatened split. When Sylvia Payne became President in the summer of 1944, she asked me to stand as Training Secretary and I was duly elected. Although still a junior member who had played no part in training, she believed I could be useful in an administrative capacity, and she also knew I shared her outlook on the need for unity. In this role, which I occupied from 1944–47, I took part in the construction of the two parallel training programmes which enabled both groups, together with the numerous Independents, to participate in training. In achieving this, great credit goes to Sylvia Payne whose fair dealing and deep concern for the future of psychoanalysis earned the respect and trust of all parties.

A fortunate fall-out of my attendance at meetings was a chance encounter with James Strachey who had taken over the editorship of the *International Journal* from Ernest Jones. In the winter of 1943–44 he remarked that he had absolutely nothing for the 1944 volume and wondered if I had anything suitable. I replied that I had rather a long paper on delinquent children which might be suitable. The upshot was that I worked every spare hour revising the draft of "Forty-Four Juvenile Thieves", (Bowlby, 1944) with valuable advice from Eric Trist. It appeared in two parts during the year and created sufficient interest that I arranged for it to be reprinted as a separate monograph. The 1500 copies, dated 1946, were sold out fairly quickly.

At the end of the war, one option for me was to start an analytic practice with a view to becoming a training analyst. Instead, I preferred to take a full-time post at the Tavistock, soon to become part of the National Health Service in charge of the Department for Children and Parents and Deputy to the Director of the Clinic, Jock Sutherland. From 1946 to 1949 I was busy recruiting staff and organizing clinical services and training courses. Amongst others, I appointed Esther Nusia Bick, a Polish psychologist who had come to England before the war and had been in analysis with Michael Balint, and who might thus be expected, once qualified, to be an Independent. She fairly soon transferred to Melanie Klein, however, and in due course became one of Mrs. Klein's most devoted disciples. This made for difficulties, especially for the child psychotherapy course which we had jointly launched in 1949, intending it to be representative of the prewar London psychoanalytic outlook, combining Independent and Kleinian orientations, and thus complementary to the course Anna Freud was organizing at the Hampstead Clinic. As time went on, however, Nusia

Bick's missionary zeal led the course to become strongly Kleinian, a shift I was unable to stop owing to my many other responsibilities. Throughout the 1950's the Kleinians were extending their grip on the Tavistock, which I regretted, since they were not interested in research.

Aspects of Melanie Klein's work which I always valued were her belief in the infant's very early capacity to make relationships and the emphasis she put on loss, mourning and depression. Her theories regarding early phases of development and the role of a death instinct struck me as implausible, however, and I was appalled by her lack of attention to a child's real-life experiences (though in that she was not alone). Since, however, there were no agreed methods of deciding between the merits of Kleinian theory and of theories held by analysts of other schools, it seemed to me necessary to be tolerant of diverse opinions. Unfortunately tolerance was never part of Melanie Klein's outlook. Certain that she possessed the truth, she looked on those who did not share her views as deplorably blind. A very insecure person, she surrounded herself with disciples whose role was not only to reassure her, but to protect her against all criticism by means of strong attack. This made discussion impossible and also led to bad feeling.

Before the war I had decided to focus my research on the effects on personality development of major disruptions in a child's relationship to his mother during the early years. Although by no means the commonest type of pathogenic experience to which a child might be exposed, it seemed to me to have three main research advantages. First, occurrence of the experience could be documented with some confidence, in contrast to disturbed relationships within the family which at that time there were no methods for study. Secondly, some long separations were outside the control of parents. This avoided our being accused of scapegoating parents, an accusation arising from misunderstanding but nonetheless frequently made. Thirdly, if the effects of gross disruptions were as serious as we believed, there were prospects of effective preventive action. Limiting our focus of research in this way proved wise, although it often led to allegations that we neglected other variables.

In two articles published in recent years[3] I have given some account of the research programme I initiated in 1949, the various publications to which it led, and the way the field has developed. Eager though I was to press forward with research which I saw as necessary if competing theories are to be evaluated, I had many other duties. Thus, I always spent about one-third of my time treating patients, including a few whom I saw once or twice a week over periods of many years. I also began holding joint family

---

3 [Bowlby note:] "Psychoanalysis as Art and Science." (Bowlby, 1979). "Attachment and Loss: Retrospect and Prospect." (Bowlby, 1982).

interviews with children and parents, and I spent one afternoon every week in a well-baby clinic, meeting with a constantly changing group of mothers and young children, trying to help the less experienced learn from those who knew more. Moreover, I supervised clinical work, and chaired case conferences, and took clinical seminars. None of this various clinical work was regarded by me as research, but it kept me in touch with all the phenomena that psychoanalytic theory is attempting to explain.

In my 1982 paper I have described how I came to regard ethology as providing psychoanalysis with an appropriate base in evolutionary biology and how over twenty-five years (1955–1980) I laboured to formulate a new conceptual framework as an alternative to Freud's metapsychology (Bowlby, 1982). Inevitably my efforts met with a mixed reception.

Throughout the nineteen-fifties I was an active member of the British Psychoanalytical Society, attending scientific meetings, at times a member of Council and for four years (1956–57 and 1958–61) Deputy President to Donald Winnicott and responsible for everything administrative. In 1952 James Robertson and I presented his film *A Two-Year-Old Goes to Hospital* (Bowlby et al., 1952) and later I presented some of the ethological findings I thought of relevance to clinical theory. Eventually in July 1957 I presented the first of a series of theoretical papers "The Nature of the Child's Tie to His Mother", (Bowlby, 1958).

Robertson's film stimulated a great deal of interest. Anna Freud, with whom he had worked in the Hampstead Nurseries, was a great enthusiast. On practical matters she and I always saw eye to eye, even if we differed on theory. The only criticism I recall came from the Kleinians. Thus, one was sure that the child's distress was a reaction to mother being pregnant. On later occasions my ethological ideas were treated with respect but aroused no great interest. The crunch came when I presented the child's tie paper, (Bowlby, 1958). I had shown a copy to a friend beforehand and, without my knowing, it had been passed to members of the Kleinian group. A number of them spoke in the discussion, criticising adversely first one aspect then another. Other members treated my ideas with respect but with no great enthusiasm.

During 1957–58 I was a fellow at the Center for Advanced Study in the Behavioral Sciences at Stanford, California – a very valuable year when I read or re-read a great deal of psychoanalytic literature and clarified for myself where I stood in relation to traditional ideas. I also gave the child's tie paper (Bowlby, 1958) in San Francisco and Los Angeles where reactions were little more favourable than in London. Amongst several friends I made that year were David and Beatrice (Betty) Hamburg. Both had been training in analysis in Chicago, but were open to many different ideas, including the possible light to be thrown on human psychology by field studies of monkeys and apes: subsequently they have been close friends and strong supporters of my efforts.

Although an innovator is always apt to recall most readily the hostile criticisms he has met with, and I am no exception, I must emphasise that I have always had strong and discriminating support from a small circle of friends and colleagues. They have read drafts, have drawn my attention to errors and ambiguities and have given me help of all kinds. Not many have been qualified analysts but all were well disposed to the orientation. Amongst those not already mentioned are Robert Hinde, who tutored me in ethology and did some critical experiments with rhesus monkeys, Mary Ainsworth who applied and elaborated my ideas in her classic study of the development of patterns of attachment during the first year, and Colin Parkes whose sensitive studies of bereaved people have greatly increased our knowledge of patterns of mourning. Among other clinicians, two family psychiatrists, Marion Mackenzie, a qualified analyst, and Dorothy Heard,[4] have been unfailing in their interest and encouragement.

Whilst at Stanford I drafted another three papers which were worked up after my return. The one on separation anxiety[5] was presented to the British Society and came in for a hostile reception from the Klein group and only limited support from elsewhere. Discussion was so brisk, however, that two further meetings were necessary for all who wished to contribute and for me to reply. Subsequent papers on mourning and its pathology were given to various psychoanalytic societies and other groups, mostly in the United States, during the early 1960s. Although they were well attended and the response of the audiences lively, my approach was too unfamiliar for more than a handful to grasp what I was attempting: and so long as I was dealing only with basic theory, the therapeutic implications, which clinicians are mainly concerned with, remained unclear. One rather typical response came from a colleague at the Tavistock: "John, we all think you have done wonderful work for children but it has nothing to do with psycho-analysis".

The upshot was that I took no further initiative in trying to communicate with my psychoanalytic colleagues. Nevertheless, I remained on good terms with them and made a point of accepting any invitation I received. One that I was especially pleased about was to be the 1980 Freud Memorial Visiting Professor of Psychoanalysis at University College London. My inaugural lecture "Psychoanalysis as a Natural Science" was published in *The International Review of Psychoanalysis* the following year (Bowlby, 1981). In addition, I gave papers and named lectures to many other audiences – psychiatrists, psychologists,

4 [Editors' note:] See Heard et al. (2009). *Attachment Therapy with Adolescents and Adults: Theory and Practice Post Bowlby.*
5 [Editors' note:] J. Bowlby (1960).

psychotherapists, social workers and ethologists. Invitations from student societies always got priority since students are likely to be less committed to traditional ideas than their elders and, in any case, theirs is the future.

Throughout the years 1964–79 I was pushing on with what, to my surprise, was to prove to be a three-volume work.[6] This detailed exposition was necessary, I thought, to avoid the new ideas being lost in the complex tangle of existing theory. (The faint-hearted may be relieved to know that any volume can be read independently of the others). Although I had sketched out most of the ground in the series of papers drafted during the previous seven years, it was only whilst I was working on these volumes that my ideas fell firmly into place. Thereafter, I became much more confident in my clinical work, including supervisions and clinical seminars.

Many analysts and other psychotherapists do excellent work using their intuition and without very clear ideas on theory, and often, I believe, in spite of the theories they nominally subscribe to, I have not that sort of mind, nor am I strong on intuition. Instead, I tend to apply such theories as I hold in an effort to understand my patient's problems. This works well when the theories are applicable but can be a big handicap when they are not. Perhaps my saving graces have been that I am a good listener and not too dogmatic about theory. As a result several of my patients have succeeded in teaching me a great deal I did not know and have contributed greatly to my understanding of different patterns of family interaction and their effects on personality development. I often shudder to think how inept I have often been as a therapist and how I have ignored or misunderstood material a patient has presented. Clearly, the best therapy is done by a therapist who is both naturally intuitive and also guided by appropriate theory. Fortunately, nowadays I meet many such people in clinical seminars and among supervisees.

Of recent years there has been a surge of interest in attachment theory by psychotherapists of diverse schools, and this is heartening. Nevertheless, since my theoretical work has always been directed primarily to my psychoanalytic colleagues in the International Association, it has been disappointing that so few, relatively, have taken notice. It has seemed to me, however, that many have been influenced, more perhaps than they have realised. Moreover, some of the younger members with a concern for science have recognised the strengths of the framework proposed. Time only, and a great deal of further research, will tell whether it proves as promising as some believe or is merely leading to a blind alley. That is the way of science.

---

6 [Editors' note:] Bowlby, J. (1969). *Attachment and Loss.* Vol. 1. *Attachment.* Bowlby, J. (1973). *Attachment and Loss. Vol. 2. Separation, Anxiety and Anger.* Bowlby, J. (1980). *Attachment and Loss. Vol. 3. Loss, Sadness and Depression.*

References

Bowlby, J. (1940). The influence of early environment in the development of neurosis and neurotic character. *International Journal of Psychoanalysis, 21*, 154–178.

Bowlby, J. (1944). Forty-four juvenile thieves: Their characters and home-life. *The International Journal of Psychoanalysis, 25*: 19–53.

Bowlby, J. (1958). The nature of the child's tie to his mother. *The International Journal of Psycho-Analysis, 39*: 350–373.

Bowlby, J. (1960). Separation anxiety. *The International Journal of Psycho-Analysis, 41*: 89–113.

Bowlby, J. (1969). *Attachment and Loss. Vol. 1. Attachment.* New York: Basic Books.

Bowlby, J. (1973). *Attachment and Loss. Vol. II. Separation: Anxiety and Anger.* New York: Basic Books.

Bowlby, J. (1979). Psychoanalysis as art and science. *The International Review of Psycho-Analysis, 6*: 3–14.

Bowlby, J. (1980). *Attachment and Loss. Vol. III. Loss, Sadness and Depression.* New York: Basic Books.

Bowlby, J. (1981). Psychoanalysis as a natural science. *The International Review of Psycho-Analysis, 8*: 243–256.

Bowlby, J. (1982). Attachment and loss: Retrospect and prospect. *American Journal of Orthopsychiatry, 52*: 664–678.

Bowlby, J., Robertson, J., & Rosenbluth, D. (1952). A Two-Year-Old Goes to Hospital. *The Psycho-Analytic Study of the Child, 7*: 82–94.

Dicks, H. V. (1970). *Fifty Years of the Tavistock Clinic.* London: Routledge & Kegan Paul.

Heard, D., Lake, B., & McCluskey, U. (2009). *Attachment Therapy with Adolescents and Adults: Theory and Practice Post-Bowlby.* London: Karnac.

Levy, D. M. (1937). Primary affect hunger. *The American Journal of Psychiatry, 94*: 643–652.

Index